HEALTH CARE LAW AND ETHICS

IN A NUTSHELL

Second Edition

By

MARK A. HALL
Professor of Law and Public Health
Wake Forest University

IRA MARK ELLMAN
Professor of Law
Arizona State University

DANIEL S. STROUSE
Professor of Law
Arizona State University

WEST
GROUP

ST. PAUL, MINN.
1999

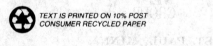

TEXT IS PRINTED ON 10% POST
CONSUMER RECYCLED PAPER

For Diana, whose constant support made this
book possible

M.A.H.

For Noah and Avi, who didn't make
it impossible

I.M.E.

For Nancy and Isabel, who make
everything possible.

D.S.S.

*

PREFACE

The content of law and medicine courses has changed dramatically in the past two decades in law schools as well as in schools of medicine, public health, and health care administration. At one time such courses were dominated by the subject of medical malpractice. This subject remains important, and is the topic of another book in the Nutshell series. But it is no longer the sole or even the dominant topic of what is now usually called health care law. The new health care law courses generally focus on one of two areas: the corporate, regulatory, and financial structure of health care delivery, and bioethics. It is these two areas that this book addresses. The increasing importance of both subjects is due in part to the incredible advances in medical technology in the decades since World War II. These advances have had two subsidiary effects. One is a phenomenal increase in the cost of health care. Because doctors can now routinely do so much more for their patients, the cost of medicine has skyrocketed, fueled in part by the development of dramatic new technologies such as organ transplants, kidney dialysis, and open heart surgery. These same medical advances also generate many additional ethical problems, for we did not confront the question of a whether a patient's life should be extended by kidney dialysis or open heart surgery before those technologies became available.

Part I of this book contains foundational chapters that are relevant to any course in health care law. It capsules the legal and policy issues of health care funding and access, and explores the legal structure and content of the doctor-patient relationship. The dramatic growth of health care spending and efforts to contain spending lead to both innovations and tensions in the business of health care. Part II addresses the legal issues that result from these structural and economic forces. Part III moves from these "macro" issues to the ethical dilemmas that arise in individual patient decisions, and covers most of the topics addressed by law school courses in bioethics.

Most schools teach the financial and structural issues of health care delivery in a separate course from the bioethical puzzles, often through different instructors. This book's first two authors have themselves followed that pattern. Other instructors, such as this book's third author, are more generalists who combine elements of both these areas with the traditional medical malpractice topics into a successful overview course. To maximize our respective talents, we have divided primary authorship responsibilities along these same lines (Hall—Chapters 1, 3, 4 and 5; Ellman—Chapters 7 and 8; and Strouse—Chapters 2 and 6). Working together on this book has persuaded us, however, that this tripartite field of law has many common themes that can and should be integrated into a more coherent whole. To that end this book is a small step.

MARK A. HALL
IRA MARK ELLMAN
DANIEL S. STROUSE

October 1998

*

A GLOSSARY OF TERMS AND ACRONYMS

The literature of health care law, and especially health care financing, is filled with acronyms and specialized terminology. We have avoided these where possible, but they are sometimes necessary, for many concepts and agencies are better known by their acronym or specialized phrase than by their full name. To ease the burden on the reader new to the subject, the following list gathers the major acronyms and terms of art used in this book primarily in first five chapters:

AMA: American Medical Association.

AHA: American Hospital Association.

CON: Certificate of Need

DHHS: U.S. Department of Health & Human Services

DRGs: Diagnosis–Related Groups—The reimbursement method recently adopted by Medicare, which pays hospitals a single, preset amount for each patient admitted according to the patient's diagnosis, age, and condition.

ERISA: Employee Retirement Income Security Act of 1974—A federal statute that primarily regulates private pension plans, but also encompasses other employee benefits such as health insurance. It has tremendous importance for the regulation of health care delivery because of a sweeping provision that preempts many traditional sources of state law.

HMO: Health Maintenance Organization—A health care organization that combines insurance and treatment functions in the same entity by providing all needed care for a lump sum annual payment.

HCFA: Health Care Financing Administration —The agency within DHHS with direct responsibility over Medicare and Medicaid.

IDS: Integrated Delivery System—Any one of a number of innovative techniques for combining hospital, physician, and insurance components into a single structure or organization.

IPA: Individual Practice Association—A form of HMO that provides care through contracting physicians who maintain independent practices in their individual offices. This structure contrasts with group HMO models in which physician owners or employees operate out of a clinic-based setting.

JCAHO: The Joint Commission on Accreditation of Healthcare Organizations—A private credentialing organization with enormous influence on hospital structure and functioning.

Managed Care: Any system of health service payment or delivery arrangements in which the health plan or provider attempts to control or coordinate health service use to contain health expenditures, improve quality, or both. Arrangements often involve a defined delivery system of providers having some form of contractual relationship with the plan.

Managed Competition: A system for choosing and paying for health insurance in which subscribers have a choice among a variety of different plans, but they must pay the most or all of the difference in price between the plan they choose and the least expensive one. Insurers in turn are required to accept all applicants and to not charge sick people more. In theory, this will force insurers to compete by managing the cost of care rather than on their ability to select only the best risks.

PHO: Physician–Hospital Organization—Any one of a number of different types of joint ventures between hospitals and physicians, usually intended as a contracting vehicle for forming a managed care network.

PPO: Preferred Provider Organization—A hybrid between traditional indemnity insurance and HMOs, in which subscribers still have a choice of physicians and providers are still paid fee-for-service, but subscribers are encouraged through financial incentives to use a select group of providers in a network, and providers agree to accept discounted payment. Similar to a point-of-service (POS) plan, which has the same elements but is licensed as a type of HMO that allows subscribers to go outside the network by paying higher deductibles and copayments.

PPS: Prospective Payment System—Another description of Medicare DRGs, one that emphasizes the fixed, preset nature of payment.

PSO: Provider Service Organization—Yet another new acronym that has cropped up recently, this one to describe an integrated delivery system headed by doctors or hospitals rather than an insurer.

RBRVS: Resource–Based Relative Value Scale—A fee schedule used by Medicare to pay physicians, which is based on the skill and effort required for each service rather than on historical billing patterns.

OUTLINE

PART II. THE LEGAL STRUCTURE OF HEALTH CARE DELIVERY

OUTLINE

TABLE OF CASES

References are to Pages

TABLE OF CASES

H

I

Q

R

S

T

U

V

TABLE OF CASES

W

HEALTH CARE LAW AND ETHICS

IN A NUTSHELL

Second Edition

*

PART I

THE FUNDAMENTALS OF HEALTH CARE DELIVERY AND FINANCE

These are exciting but challenging times in which to study health care law for it was only in the 1980s that the law began fully to confront an unprecedented shift in health care policy. Traditionally, the exclusive focus of health care policy was on advancing the state of medical science. Over the past decade, however, two new concerns have begun to dominate the health care policy agenda: the cost of and access to medical treatment. Limiting incessant inflation in health care spending for the bulk of the population covered by insurance and finding ways to afford health care coverage for the medically indigent are issues of paramount importance in the decisionmaking of law makers, medical practitioners, and health care institutions.

The fundamental reorientation in perspective caused by this shift in focus from advances to restraints and distribution demands a thorough rethinking of traditional legal doctrine from the ground up. Legal precedents rooted in the expansionist medical care system of the post-war era may no longer make sense in an era when the controlling public policy is to limit or allocate governmental and private health care spending. For example, perhaps malpractice law should take account of the economic costs as well as the medical risks of treatment decisions. Or perhaps antitrust, tax and corporate law should be more lenient about how medical institutions are structured and operated. In the field of bioethics, perhaps the law has gone too far in allowing physicians to withdraw care without regard to patients' wishes.

So that the reader may acquire a deeper understanding of these new legal challenges, Chapter 1 explores the policy and economic environment that shapes the agenda for contemporary health care law and ethics. Chapter 2 then looks at the areas of legal doctrine that directly affect a patient's right to receive health care, and the structure and content of the doctor-patient relationship.

CHAPTER 1

HEALTH INSURANCE COVERAGE AND REGULATORY REFORM

A. THE CRISIS IN HEALTH CARE SPENDING AND COVERAGE

1. The Dimensions of the Crisis

a. The Spending Crisis

An astounding rate of inflation has gripped the American health care system over the past four decades. Per capita medical costs have increased 2000 percent since 1960, a rate of increase that has doubled expenditures about every six years. We now spend a trillion dollars annually on health care, which is about 14 percent of the gross national product. As startling as the present day facts are, these trends are even more disturbing considering the prolongation of life spans and the vast increase in elderly population that will occur with the aging of the baby boom generation.

These increases in spending might be celebrated as a great American success story if we believed they produced commensurable benefits. After all, nothing is more treasured than our health; why shouldn't we spend as much as possible to enhance it? There are three responses to this observation. First, all spending is inherently a trade-off because we can always spend on something else instead. While our health is surely an important priority, it simply is not true that people always treat health as more important than competing values. We see this every day, not only when we smoke, drink, or eat excessively, but also when we drive to work or we read a book rather than exercise. Second, even if we focus on our health as the overriding value, we must realize that there are other ways to promote health than through medical care. In the words of one prominent health policy analyst, "once a reasonable minimum level of care is provided, factors other than medical care—diet, lifestyle, heredity, environment—appear to have much more effect on health and longevity than does more or less medical care. Above a reasonable minimum, the availability of more medical care resources appears to have little or no effect on many indicators of health status." A. Enthoven, Health Plan xvi (1980). In other words, we are likely to produce greater health bang for the buck by spending less on medicine and more on nutrition, shelter, the environment, education to improve lifestyles and other preventive measures.

The idea that American medicine is an unqualified success story is also undermined by international comparisons. We spend substantially more per capita and devote much more of our GDP to health care than any other peer nation. Our spending is 50–to–100 percent higher than most industrialized countries, and 2–to–3 times higher than some, such as England. At the same time, the U.S. ranks near the bottom in major indicators of health status such as life expectancy at birth and infant mortality. To some extent, this is due to social factors that create health problems. By other indicators American medicine is the best in the world. For instance, the chance of dying once a person has a major disease is much lower in America than other countries. Still, it appears that Americans are not getting the same bang for their medical buck as are other countries. It has been documented that much of what we spend on medical care is simply waste, yielding no benefit of any kind. Examples of unnecessary care proliferate throughout American medicine:

> Studies indicate that at least 25% of the money we spend on health care is wasted.... Hospitals operate at an average of two-thirds of their capacity, with many at less than 50%. We have up to 400,000 excess hospital beds, at an unnecessary cost of up to $12 billion. We also suffer from excess technology. There are 10,000 mammography machines in operation, four times the number actually needed.... Millions of unnecessary procedures and tests are performed each year. Almost half the coronary bypasses, the majority of Caesarean sections, and a significant proportion of many other procedures, such as pacemaker implants and carotid endarterectomies, are unnecessary or of questionable value. A former editor of the Journal of the American

Medical Association is convinced that more than half of the forty million medical tests performed each day "do not really contribute to a patient's diagnosis or therapy." Doctors order many procedures and tests to protect themselves from potential medical malpractice liability. Some procedures are performed because doctors simply do not know the precise circumstances under which many procedures work.

Joseph A. Califano, Rationing Health Care: The Unnecessary Solution, 140 U. Pa. L. Rev. 1525 (1992).

b. *The Coverage Crisis*

Medical inflation is not the only health care crisis gripping our country. We are also facing a crisis of epidemic proportions in health insurance coverage. At the same time that we have devoted massive resources to the health care of most of our populace, we have largely ignored the health care needs of a significant segment of our society. The ranks of the medically indigent have increased dramatically to the point that an estimated 40 million people (almost 20 percent of those under age 65) are uninsured at any point in time.

This situation exists because many employers do not offer their workers private health insurance as a job benefit, especially smaller employers and those that hire seasonal and temporary workers. Workers without insurance can buy individual coverage, but that is more expensive than group coverage, and these workers often have low-wage jobs or are young and healthy and so do not perceive the need for health insurance.

The gaps in private insurance are partially filled by two major public programs, Medicaid and Medicare, but Medicaid covers only those who are poor and Medicare covers the elderly or disabled. Medicare is reasonably comprehensive. Almost everyone who is over 65 and retired is eligible, and those who aren't can buy in for a reasonable fee. But Medicaid falls far short of its objective. It covers less than half of people falling below the federal poverty guidelines. This results from two factors. First, Medicaid is a joint program between state and federal governments, and individual states have discretion to set the income guidelines where they wish. Second, federal rules restrict Medicaid eligibility to specified categories of poverty that attempt to define who are the "deserving poor." Simple poverty does not suffice in most states; one must also be elderly, disabled, or the parent of a dependent child. These are the traditional categories covered by welfare. Moreover, observe that most people without insurance are not poor by traditional criteria. They or their family members work in low-wage jobs that provide no insurance. When they are ill, they must either pay out of pocket, go to publicly-funded clinics and hospitals which are sparsely located and woefully underfunded, or seek charitable care from hospitals, usually in the emergency room.

Coverage is even more deficient for certain categories of care. Many well-insured workers have little or no coverage of mental health treatment or long-term care in nursing homes. Long-term care is an issue of special concern as the ranks of the very old are beginning to escalate. Traditional health insurance, including Medicare, covers nursing home and home health care only for short periods of time. Long-term care of this nature requires separate insurance, which most people do not think to purchase until they need it, which makes the price not worth it or too high to afford for most people. Some can afford to pay for care out of pocket, but the only fall-back for many people is Medicaid. A major portion of Medicaid funding goes to cover the costs of nursing home care for the middle class elderly. These people qualify by first "spending down" their available wealth on the first few years of nursing care and, once impoverished, then going onto Medicaid. For a time, careful estate planning could produce the same result by transferring wealth to trusts or to family members, but a series of statutory amendments have virtually eliminated the ability to qualify without actually spending down to below the poverty line.

2. The Causes of the Spending Crisis

The two dimensions of the present crisis in health care spending—inflation and lack of coverage—are thought to be related. In the public financing sphere, we have great difficulty extending comprehensive coverage to everyone precisely because the level of spending under current programs has proven to be uncontrollable. In the private sphere, many low-wage employees fail to receive health insurance through their jobs because the level of care that most of us have come to expect (and hence that the private insurance market offers) is so extravagant. Therefore, the first task of health care policy is to understand the causes and possible solutions to the relentless inflation that has gripped health care spending over the past generation. After that, we will look at proposals for making access to health insurance more comprehensive.

a. The Structure of Traditional Insurance

Health policy analysts agree that the central cause of the uncontrolled increase in health care spending is the "complex of irrational economic incentives" inherent in our conventional health insurance system. A. Enthoven *supra* at 16. Some three-fourths of medical treatment is funded by third-party payers—either private insurance policies available primarily through employment or government programs available to the elderly and poor. Traditionally, *private* insurance—such as that available through Blue Cross and Blue Shield—has been structured on a piece-work basis known as "fee-for-service," whereby doctors and hospitals are paid a separate amount for each discrete item of service. The structure of traditional *government* reimbursement—such as the Medicare program—has been cost-based (for hospitals) or charge-based (for doctors), whereby providers are reimbursed for most of their costs or charges incurred in treating covered patients. These traditional forms of reimbursement create a host of powerful cost-escalating incentives that affect each actor in the health care system.

b. The Incentives for Patients

The patient has virtually no incentive to economize under this system of insurance. Because a third party is footing most of the bill, patients are eager to receive (and have now come to expect and demand) all care that is of any conceivable benefit. In economic terminology, this tendency of insurance to induce disregard of costs is known as a form of "moral hazard" (analogous to the incentive that a well-insured warehouse owner might have to avoid taking precautions against fire). Although it is debatable whether well-insured patients may be less concerned about taking preventive measures, it is indisputable that traditional insurance induces them to order more treatment than they otherwise would when they do fall ill or suffer an accident.

One might expect insured patients to scrutinize medical expenditures in order to avoid future premium increases. This is one deterrent to careless driving under auto insurance, for example. The reason this cost-internalization safeguard does not work is the lack of "experience rating" in health insurance. Rather than individualizing premiums to the specific medical treatment record of particular patients (as auto insurers do for drivers), health insurers historically engaged in "community rating," a system that charges the same for everyone in the insurance pool. Blue Cross/Blue Shield, the largest network of health insurers, was notable in this regard. Other insurers, while individualizing premiums to some extent, still use large groups of employees as their basis for setting group rates. Even to the extent that health insurance is experience rated, *patients* still are not likely to realize the financial impact of their treatment decisions since the great bulk of insurance is provided in the employment setting. Therefore, the employer is the one who picks up the tab for insurance premium increases. Moreover, the fact that employer-paid insurance premiums are not taxed as income to the employee creates a strong tax incentive for employees to prefer lower wages over being required to pay a portion of the premium themselves.

Another way to describe this set of incentives is through the economic concept of the "free rider" effect. Because the costs of treatment decisions are not internalized to the patient but instead are spread to others in the employee group or the community, individual patients are able to take a free ride when they spend excessively. This effect is most pronounced under government insurance, where the costs of treatment are financed through the general tax base and therefore borne by society at large.

"[O]ne wonders what people thought *would* control cost in such a system. One of the main answers is deductibles and coinsurance. Make the patient pay the first $200 of each year's medical bills and 25 percent of the cost above that, and he will be

cost-conscious and go to the doctor only when necessary.... This principle has been applied in most
health insurance in the United States." A. Enthoven, Health Plan 32–33 (1980). This cost-sharing
principle has not worked well for several reasons.
First, cost-sharing is not universal. Under labor
union pressure, many employers during the past
generation turned to "first-dollar" coverage that
eliminated all cost to the patient. Second, even
where the patient shares some of the costs, she
realizes and incorporates into her decisionmaking
only the portion of the costs she bears. Consider
how our eating habits would differ if we had to pay
only one-quarter of the costs of our food.

Even to the extent that patients do realize the
costs of treatment, an additional barrier to cost
consciousness arises from the fact that most people
delegate medical decisions to their doctors because
they lack the knowledge and expertise to compe-
tently evaluate their doctors' treatment recommendations. It is a perverse market that places purchasing decisions in the hands of sellers rather than
buyers, but this phenomenon of "supplier-induced
demand" is what characterizes the traditional market for health care services. Thus, as a generaliza-
tion, it is probably more accurate to view the health
care system as driven by the decisions of physicians
than by those of patients. For this reason, it becomes critical to understand the set of incentives
that traditional reimbursement creates for health
care providers.

c. The Incentives for Providers

To the extent that physicians control treatment decisions, the third-party character of insurance—the fact that someone else is footing the bill—results in a lack of cost consciousness in health care purchasing decisions, reinforcing the economically absurd "spare-no-expense" philosophy just described. But this is not the entire story. Traditional insurance is riddled with other incentives that are equally or more perverse with respect to physician behavior. Primarily, the particular structure of the payments made under traditional insurance—fee-for-service or cost/charge-based—has a critical influence on medical practice. Under fee-for-service reimbursement, doctors and hospitals are paid more the more they treat. This "piece work" payment method has three results: First, it exacerbates the "spare-no-expense" ethic described above to the extent that providers have an incentive to render not only all care that has any benefit, but also care that may be of *no* benefit (or only of very uncertain benefit). Second, fee-for-service reimbursement deemphasizes preventive care, which is usually not as lucrative for providers. Third, this payment system encourages an excessive reliance on medical technology by paying for discrete procedures rather than for the time spent with patients and by encouraging the medicalization of social problems. Traditional insurance has thus been blamed for the current ills of overspecialization, excessive reliance on inpatient hospitalization, and triple-teaming cases.

The problems of fee-for-service reimbursement are aggravated by the way in which the fee is set. Traditionally, both private and government insurers have allowed doctors to charge whatever the market will bear, and, since there has been no effective market restraint, this has meant paying doctors whatever they ask for. The acronym for this practice is "UCR" payment—"usual, customary and reasonable." Hospitals have been equally profligate under the cost-based payment system that prevails for their services. As further detailed in section A.2.e, which discusses traditional Medicare reimbursement, reimbursing hospitals for the full costs of treatment rewards them for extravagant services.

This is not to say that doctors and hospitals act only out of economic motives. Indeed, providers may not even consciously consider the economic implications of their actions. Nevertheless, the economic environment created by third-party, fee-for-service, charge/cost based reimbursement certainly facilitates and reinforces an inflationary practice style. It is impossible to expect doctors to be impervious to these fundamental economic forces. Indeed, it might be considered unethical for doctors to act in any other way. Ethicists maintain that a doctor's fiduciary duty to his patients requires him to act solely with the patient's interests in mind. If costs are of no consequence to the patient, then they should not enter into the doctor's calculus. *See* R. Veatch, A Theory of Medical Ethics 158 (1981). But if costs are of no consequence to the patient or the doctor, then who will insist upon efficiency and value in medical expenditures? This oversight role is left to third parties—employers and insurers (both private and government).

d. The Incentives for Insurers and Employers

In a system of third-party reimbursement funded by employers and the government, both they and the insurers have strong incentives to restrain costs. Yet, several dynamics within the health care system have made it difficult for third parties to impose meaningful discipline. First, the prevalence of the "free choice of provider" principle kept insurers from using competitive bidding to impose cost discipline on the medical profession or the hospital industry. Organized medicine has campaigned heavily throughout the 20th century to give patients the freedom to select any doctor or hospital they desire while maintaining comprehensive insurance. Some commentators argue that this ostensible consumer choice ethic has been misused to achieve anticompetitive ends, because requiring insurers to reimburse all providers in full eliminates any opportunity for insurers to select relatively more efficient doctors or hospitals through a competitive bidding process. *See* Charles Weller, *"Free Choice" as a Restraint of Trade in American Health Care Delivery,* 69 Iowa L.Rev. 1351 (1984).

Private and government insurers might attempt to regulate provider behavior by rigorous scrutiny of the need for medical services through the process of individual claims review. Such "utilization review" techniques face the obstacle of developing acceptable methods for identifying unnecessary care, a task made difficult by the fact that only a very small portion of medical care is of a life-or-death nature. The vast bulk of medical decisions are focused on questions such as whether an extra diagnostic test or an extra day in the hospital is worthwhile, questions to which there are no clear answers. At the margin, it is extremely difficult to say that a particular item of service has no benefit whatsoever. It is even more difficult to say when a procedure is not worth its cost if it has *some* benefit.

Such assessments are rendered impossible in part by the extent of uncertainty in medical knowledge. This uncertainty results in large part from the difficulty of conducting elaborate controlled studies to test the relative benefits of all the many options available to treat each medical condition. Without a firm, scientific basis on which to critique medical decisionmaking, insurers are forced as a practical matter to acquiesce in a system that allows the very persons who are receiving reimbursement to exercise the sole authority over certifying the legitimacy of the expenditures. Even if dispositive studies were available, physician oversight would be deterred by the intensely judgmental nature of medical practice. This notion is captured in the slogan that medical practice is more an art than a science, meaning that physicians' treatment decisions are guided more by soft, subjective reasoning processes than by rigorous, deductive logic. As a result, it is difficult for someone other than the patient's personal physician to dictate the details of treatment, even if a third party's judgment were equally valid from an objective perspective. The conventional consequence of these various factors was to cede to practicing physicians nearly complete authority over treatment decisions.

e. Traditional Medicare Reimbursement

The structure of traditional Medicare reimbursement for hospitals provides an excellent microcosm of the failings of conventional insurance. Medicare, which covers the elderly and disabled regardless of wealth or income, was enacted during the liberal euphoria of the 1960s. It has two basic parts: Part A (the focus of the following discussion), covers the services of hospitals and other facilities; Part B covers physician and outpatient services.

The hospital industry and the medical profession lobbied against Medicare (and Medicaid) when these programs were in their planning stages because hospitals and doctors viewed large-scale government intrusion into medicine as a potential threat to their interests. Congress, concerned that the necessary level of cooperation would not be forthcoming, responded to this pressure by crafting Medicare with several elements favorable to providers.

Primarily, Medicare was modeled after traditional private insurance with fee-for-service payment and free choice of physician. For doctor services, Part B of Medicare pays 80 percent of "reasonable charges." Part A initially reimbursed hospital services 100 percent of the costs of treatment less a deductible and copayments. This was changed in 1983 for most hospitals, but is still the case for specialized hospitals and facilities. The particular measure of cost chosen provided ample allowance for rapid depreciation of assets and even paid profit-making hospitals an amount reflecting a return on investment. Moreover, the government decided not to undertake itself the task of administering reimbursement, instead contracting out these accounting details to "fiscal intermediaries," usually Blue Cross and Blue Shield, which are creatures of the hospital industry.

As a result of these various fundamental structural elements, Medicare expenditures quickly mushroomed far beyond initial projections. The facts of Sacred Heart Hospital v. United States, 616 F.2d 477, 479 (Ct.Cl.1980), a typical reimbursement dispute at one hospital, provide a representative illustration: "Prior to 1963, ... the [respiratory therapy] department, as such, consisted of a non-certified therapist and a technician who were trained to administer oxygen.... [Since then], the department has grown to eight full time, board certified anesthesiologists, nine trained technicians, two therapists and two registered therapists."

In addition to the problem of controlling costs, traditional hospital reimbursement under Medicare faced the problem of *measuring* costs, a formidable task given the numerous items of indirect and overhead expenses incurred in hospital treatment. The formula used by Medicare to apportion total hospital costs between government and private patients was a ratio of charges for Medicare patients to charges for private patients. However, charges do not serve as a uniform proxy for costs: the percentage mark-up can vary widely among different departments of the hospital. Hospitals therefore could manipulate their charge structures to overbill Medicare, for instance, by marking up surgery charges (which are more heavily used by Medicare patients) by 50 percent while marking up obstetrics charges (rarely used by Medicare patients) by only 25 percent. To correct for this manipulative pricing behavior, it was necessary to apply the ratio of Medicare charges to total charges within each department of the hospital. Still, hospitals were free to manipulate their pricing structures within each department.

Finally, traditional Medicare reimbursement has proven extremely complex in its administrative and judicial review process. Discussion of the Medicare appeals process would be too lengthy for this book, but suffice it to say that courts and regulators are continually plagued by constitutional, statutory, and administrative law controversies over the proper timing, process and scope of review of various Medicare decisions.

f. *Managed Care and the Structure of Health Insurance*

Considering that the structure of health insurance lies at the root of so many of these economic and social problems, it makes sense to ask why this structure dominated for so many decades. Medical sociologist Paul Starr and other scholars have documented a sustained and enormously successful campaign by organized medicine to suppress or coopt alternative insurance models that would have been more threatening to its economic interests. *See, e.g.,* Paul Starr, The Social Transformation of American Medicine 226 (1982). Generally, "of the variety of insurance structures that might have taken shape, the predominant model, indemnity, was one that did not intervene in doctors' relationships with patients or hospitals and did not interfere with their style of practice. Physicians suppressed ... other financing models that would have placed doctors in a more subordinate position, models such as direct benefit insurance epitomized by the modern HMO.... The Great Society programs of the 1960s reflect the continuing institutional accommodation of physician interests. Cowed by fears of physician and hospital boycotts, lawmakers infused Medicare and Medicaid with a number of highly favorable structural elements patterned on the prevailing private insurance model. The dominating protectionist influence is codified in the programs' first words, which guarantee freedom from 'any supervision or control over the practice of medicine or the manner in which medical services are provided.' "Mark A. Hall, *Institutional Control of Physician Behavior: Legal Barriers to Health Care Cost Containment,* 137 U.Pa.L.Rev. 431, 446 (1988). *See also* S. Law, Blue Cross: What Went Wrong (2d ed. 1976).

For these reasons, most attempts to solve the spending crisis are aimed at one or more of the traditional structural features. The next section describes these reforms in more detail, but it is useful to lay the groundwork here by describing the phenomenon of managed care. Much of this section has been or could be stated in the past tense since traditional insurance structures are giving way so rapidly to various components of managed care. These components are embodied to different degrees in the specific forms of insurance described below (HMOs, PPOs, DRGs, etc.), but it is possible to abstract from these particulars the three general features of managed care. Each responds to a key feature of traditional insurance. HMOs embody all three components to the fullest extent.

First, managed care erodes the free choice of physician principle by contracting selectively with doctors and hospitals to form a network of providers, and then controlling movement within the network through "gatekeeping" physicians. HMOs require that subscribers enroll with a primary care physician in the network, who they must first consult in order to receive referrals to designated specialists. PPOs and point of service plans allow patients to go outside the network by paying higher deductibles and copayments.

The second feature is more intensive utilization review. No longer does insurance cover virtually anything a physician orders. Prior approval must be obtained from the insurer before initiating an expensive course of treatment. The third managed care feature is payment incentives. Rather than pay physicians and hospitals on a piece-work basis,

HMOs and other insurers use payment incentives that reward providers for saving treatment costs.

At present, almost everyone with public or private insurance is subject to one or more of these managed care components. In other words, pure unconstrained fee-for-service indemnity insurance is virtually extinct. Nevertheless, important aspects of the traditional structure are still widespread and worth preserving, and it is still the case that less than half the insured population belongs to HMOs. To understand how we have moved so quickly from the old to the new, and where this transition may eventually be heading, the next section systematically reviews a variety of reform proposals that have been considered or pursued. We begin first with reforms that seek to expand insurance coverage, and then consider reforms aimed as saving costs.

B. INSURANCE COVERAGE REFORM

There is a broad spectrum of reform ideas intended to increase insurance coverage, which range from the most to the least government involvement. None of these have been implemented in their purest form, nor have any been completely rejected. In our complex and fragmented system, each exists to some extent and in an imperfect or compromised form. But looking at each in isolation helps to dissect the anatomy of our current system and to understand how it might be reconfigured. This also is a good opportunity to learn more about how insurance is structured in other countries to which reformers look for their models.

1. Socialized Medicine and the British System

The AMA often attacks reform ideas as socialized medicine, thinking that government take-over of the health care system lurks around virtually every corner. But seldom does anyone actually propose true socialized medicine. The purest example comes from the British National Health Service ("NHS"), where the government owns and operates the entire health care delivery system and guarantees comprehensive coverage to all of its citizens. This is generally considered to be a completely un-American approach, in view of the multitude of differences that exist between our two societies in political structures, cultural attitudes, and historical settings. Nevertheless, features of this approach are prominent in our current system, in the form of government hospitals. States have mental hospitals, large cities have general municipal hospitals, the Veterans Administration and the military operate a large hospital and medical system, and the Indian Health Service maintains facilities mostly on reservations.

Listing these examples is usually sufficient to defeat this as an idea for comprehensive reform. Although some of these hospitals are among the finest in the country (e.g., Bethesda Naval), many are among the worst. Looking to England, where facilities are outmoded and overcrowded, confirms

that government-run systems can be woefully underfunded. In our country, the condition and quality of government hospitals for the poor could be
vastly improved through increased funding, but as
long as they serve primarily the poor, the necessary
political constituency will always be lacking.

2. Single Payer, Canadian–Style Insurance

In contrast with socialized medicine is socialized
insurance, in which the delivery of care remains in
private hands but the government assumes the insurance or payment function. This is how the Cana-
dian system is structured, and it is the essence of
Medicare in our country. The reform proposal is to
extend Medicare to the entire country by essentially
prohibiting private insurance, resulting in a single
source of payment for all medical care. Although
Canada, like England, has long waiting lines and
underfunded facilities, this is not necessarily how
the idea would take shape in the U.S. if we were
willing to support more generous funding. The potential compatibility of this idea with American
values is demonstrated by the fact that Medicare is
widely popular with the elderly.

Two other arguments speak in favor of single-
payer reform. One looks to the savings in administrative costs. Competing private insurers generate a
significant percentage of "wasted" spending on
marketing, administration, and profits. Advocates
claim these costs could be greatly reduced or eliminated through the streamlining and economies of
scale of having a single, mandatory insurance plan.

One measure of the potential savings is to look at the "medical loss ratios" for private insurers, that is, the portion of the premium dollar they collect that goes directly to paying for treatment. For group insurance, this ranges from 70 to 90 percent, and it is even lower for individual insurance. Medicare, however, runs at a medical loss ratio in the high 90s. The 10–20 percent savings that are available might be enough by itself to pay for everyone without insurance.

The second argument is a moral one. A single-payer system promotes both vertical equity and horizontal equity. Vertical equity speaks to who contributes. Horizontal equity speaks to who is eligible and what they receive. Private insurance requires at best that everyone contribute the same amount, but at worst requires those with the greatest need to contribute the most. On the receiving end, only those who pay are eligible for private insurance and its benefits are set by the level of contribution. In contrast, public insurance entirely disconnects contribution from need and benefits. Contributions are based on the ability to pay, through the general taxation system. Benefits are determined entirely by need.

There are several compelling responses to these compelling arguments. The first is simply the pragmatic political observation that converting entirely to a single payer system would mean that the entire health insurance industry would have to close shop. It would also mean moving hundreds of billions of dollars of expenditures from the private sector onto the tax-and-spend ledgers of the government. In an era of "no new taxes," anti-entitlement programs, and eliminating the budget deficit, this large scale conversion of 1/7 of the economy is considered politically unfeasible.

The response to the administrative cost argument observes that not all these costs are wasted. Some portion goes toward holding down the costs of treatment, through managed care techniques. Another portion goes toward providing consumers more choice in the selection of insurance arrangements and benefits.

The moral argument raises the question of whether everyone should be entitled to the same level of insurance, determined entirely by need. It sounds agreeable to advocate equal access to health care, but we don't currently maintain equal access to any other fundamental social good such as housing, food, income, or education. Instead, we attempt to provide a socially adequate minimum and allow people to make private purchases above the minimum. A "two-tier" system of medicine violates some people's egalitarian moral code, but many people are willing to accept some inequity if the bottom tier is at least decent. At present, it is our insistence on state-of-the-art medicine that makes it difficult to afford any coverage for 15 percent of the population. Relaxing the egalitarian standard could make decent coverage affordable for everyone. Insisting on strict egalitarianism would violate libertarian principles by requiring that upper limits be set on the care that the wealthy are free to purchase. Therefore, most people find some differentiation in access to be morally acceptable. *See* President's Commission, Securing Access to Health Care (1983). This would mean allowing people to purchase private insurance that supplements or replaces public programs, which Canada does not allow. Medicare does allow this, but at present it discourages physicians from accepting more payment than Medicare allows, which frustrates the ability of Medicare patients to shop for the very best doctors.

3. Employer or Individual Mandates

A more realistic solution is to require all employers to provide insurance. This was the heart of President Clinton's failed proposal in 1993. To its credit, it builds on the existing and popular employer-based private system, and it achieves economies of scale by covering most people in groups. Germany has successfully achieved universal insurance through an employer mandate, as has Hawaii.

The primary objection is that increasing employers' costs will, similar to increasing the minimum wage, only hurt those we are trying to help by causing employers to eliminate a number of jobs at the margin. Another objection is that an employer mandate expands and perpetuates the distorting incentives created by exempting employer-provided insurance from personal income tax. This also neglects the self-employed.

Another alternative to consider, therefore, is an individual mandate, that is, requiring everyone to obtain their own insurance, either through employment or on their own. Uncoupling insurance from employment would remove the tax distortion and allow more choice for those who don't like the insurance their employer offers. (This would also avoid the ERISA preemption problems discussed in chapter 5.C.)

The real difficulty with either an employer or individual mandate, however, is structuring the subsidies that are necessary to make insurance purchase affordable for everyone. An employer mandate usually comes with subsidies for small employers (those with 50 or fewer workers), only half whom currently buy insurance, but attaching the subsidy to the size of firm is a poor proxy for who can really afford insurance. Many small firms are highly profitable, and many large firms have lots of low-wage workers. It is also unfair to deny subsidies to struggling firms that in the past have met their social obligation.

Subsidies for individuals are equally difficult to structure. Most people without insurance have workers in their family and are not poor, but with family coverage costing $3–5000 a year, they simply can't afford it. The government could simply raise the threshold for Medicaid eligibility, but this would create a huge disincentive to take on extra work or a better-paying job, since a few hundred dollars more of income might result in losing $1000s in benefits. So some sliding scale subsidy is necessary, in which the level of support falls more gradually as income increases. The slope would have to be quite gentle, however, in order to avoid a severe disincentive to work, since extra earnings also mean losing other social benefits and mean paying more taxes. But the slower the drop-off in subsidy, the greater the cost.

This is one of the dilemmas that undermined the 1993 Clinton health care reform proposal. The subsidies it required to make insurance affordable were so expensive that adequate funding sources could not be found. The Clinton plan attempted to hide the costs by redirecting funding from Medicare, but this incurred the wrath of the elderly. The Clinton plan tried to keep the subsidies down by severely capping the rate of increase in health insurance premiums, but that antagonized insurers and providers. Simply increasing broad-based taxes was also not politically feasible. So the plan imploded under its own weight.

4. Incremental Reforms

The lesson that lawmakers learned from the Clinton plan failure is that comprehensive health insurance reform is too complex and politically volatile to accomplish, at least in the present era. So, instead, they have turned to various ideas for incremental reform. These are attempts to shore up the places where insurance coverage is eroding the most rapidly, recognizing that this will not achieve universal coverage, but at least will move in the right direction, or will keep us from backsliding. This also builds on the current system.

Examples of this incremental approach abound, both in public and private insurance. In the public system, examples include various expansions of Medicaid to cover children and pregnant women. In the private sector, there are various state and federal laws that make it easier for employers or workers to obtain and keep coverage. One of these laws, abbreviated COBRA, requires insurers to offer employees coverage at group rates for 18 months after they leave the job. Another law, abbreviated HIPAA, requires insurers after the 18 months expire to convert this group coverage to individual coverage, but allows insurers to charge whatever they want. HIPAA, along with state laws, also prevents insurers from turning down any small employer (50 and under) who wants coverage, regardless of the health status of its workers or their families. And these same laws allow employees to switch insurers without undergoing a new pre-existing condition exclusion period, a concept known as "portability." This keeps workers with health problems from being locked into their current job. State laws (but not federal) also restrict the extent to which insurers can vary their premiums according to the health status of small employer groups. Some states require community rating for small employers.

This complicated and fragmented approach has the following limitations. First, the purchase of insurance remains voluntary and unsubsidized, so many people continue to decline to purchase. Moreover, some of these reforms may end up making insurance more costly. Community rating, for instance, attracts older, sicker subscribers and makes insurance less affordable of younger, healthier ones, a phenomenon known as "adverse selection." Therefore, only a few states require insurers to offer individual insurance at community rates to all applicants, and those that do have seen insurance premiums increase and the number of purchasers drop. More commonly, states create a high risk pool for individuals who cannot get health insurance or require Blue Cross plans to offer such insurance, but these options usually cost 50 to 100 percent more than normal market rates, which are already very expensive.

5. Managed Competition

A final set of reform ideas known as "managed competition" cuts across this spectrum of proposals. It is adaptable to many of these approaches and therefore has been implemented in a number of settings. The leading advocate is a Stanford health economist, Alain Enthoven. The essence of managed competition is a voucher concept, in which subscribers can select from a range of insurance options in both the public and the private sectors, but in a monitored market environment that encourages them to make a cost-conscious choice of the insurance that offers the best value for them. Unlike conventional Medicare and Medicaid, people would have a choice of insurance arrangements, some from the private sector. Unlike employment-based insurance, the choice would be made by the individual, not the employer. And, unlike either, the individual would bear the full marginal cost of the choice.

Managed competition proposals vary quite a bit in their detail, but they look something like this. An employer or government program would give each person a voucher that represents the full value of the cheapest available plan that offers decent coverage. The voucher amount would not vary according to the kind of insurance selected. If people pick a more expensive plan, they pay the full cost differential. They can select from any approved plan in the market, including buying into a government insurance plan. This maximizes choice and creates a strong incentive to shop for the best cost/quality trade-off. Managed competition does not necessarily equate with managed care, but it is assumed that, when faced with this choice, most people will opt for managed care.

This idea is widely adaptable. It currently is used by many large employers. Medicare was recently amended to create a new Part C (called Medicare + Choice) which will function in roughly this fashion. Purchasing cooperatives have been created in several states to bring this same vehicle to small employers. This was also a centerpiece of the Clinton plan, which would have created a nationwide system of government-run purchasing cooperatives (called Health Alliances) through which almost all insurance would be sold.

Whether this approach offers the optimal solution for structuring the insurance market remains to be seen. No idea is without potential problems. One can imagine, for instance, that difficult decisions would be faced in determining which services should be included in the set of benefits that constitutes the baseline, for these benefits would then not be subject to market choice. Would the government be able to resist pressures to require coverage of life-saving organ transplants or dramatic new innovations in diagnostic technology like MRI and PET scanners? Should it? Also, the voucher amounts would have to be adjusted to reflect the relative risk status of different subscribers, in order to counteract insurers' incentives to avoid high risks. Otherwise, insurers could profit by engaging in selective marketing or poor service to high risk subscribers. Developing an accurate risk adjustment measure that cannot be gamed is a tall task that researchers have not yet accomplished. More fundamental is the concern that people will be confused and upset by all the choices and complicated information being forced on them, especially the elderly. In sum, the "managed" component of managed competition may involve too much complexity and government oversight if the system is to run smoothly and fairly. That in essence is what doomed the Clinton proposal.

C.   INTERLUDE: ECONOMIC AND REGULATORY THEORY

The prior section reveals that two opposing political and economic theories—government regulation versus free markets—influence different approaches for increasing access to health care, and we will see in the next section that the same is true for approaches to containing costs. This section is an interlude in which we discuss the theoretical framework for reform in more detail. We begin with the premise of these reforms that limited social resources must be allocated more wisely, and we then discuss competing views on whether allocation decisions are best made by market or regulatory forces.

1. The Need for Health Care Rationing

Our starting premise is that any successful reform effort must in some measure ration health care resources, that is, set limits on spending that deny some beneficial care, and in so doing allocate the limited resources among competing treatment needs. "Rationing" may seem an excessively harsh term for this process, since allocation is inherent in society's use of *any* resource (given that all resources are limited to some degree), but explicitness is necessary here in order to shake us from the romanticism that sometimes clouds the reality that even life-saving resources are not available in endless quantities. This is a disturbing reality because Americans have come to take medical miracles for granted and have come to expect the latest technological advances to be readily available to everyone. It is hard to conceive of Americans accepting, for instance, the practice that prevails in England where patients over 55 seldom receive kidney dialysis.

The symbolic values we attach to health care are illustrated by the contradictory attitudes we take toward saving "statistical" as opposed to "identifiable" lives. Daily, our society calmly suffers great statistical human tragedies such as highway deaths and the health effects of pollution or unhealthy lifestyles that could be reduced by increased tax funding for precautionary or educational measures, but when public attention is brought to an identifiable individual suffering from a present illness— say, a small child suffering from liver failure—we respond passionately with an outpouring of donations to support even extraordinarily expensive medical treatment. When the threat is imminent, there is a strongly-felt sense of injustice in a system that would allow a preventable death to occur, but not so for probablistic risks of equal or greater magnitude. This paradox is one of the difficulties public policy makers face in engaging in more explicit health care rationing.

The need for health care rationing is better understood by viewing health care inflation as composed of two components: built-up waste and future waste. Current treatment patterns are infiltrated with instances of unnecessary care that have become ingrained in a fee-for-service practice style. We clearly need to trim the fat out of our present system, but medical science is continually producing technological advances that will quickly swamp the effect of such a one-time savings. In recent years we have seen the advent of magnetic resonance imaging and organ transplants. In the near future, we will witness the proliferation of artificial organ *im-*plants, even more exotic diagnostic machinery, and, not too far down the road, genetic therapies, all extraordinarily expensive yet promising medical advances. In order to accomplish meaningful reform, we need some measure that will both tighten our current belts and resist future temptations. Wm. Schwartz, *The Inevitable Failure of Current Cost–Containment Strategies: Why They Can Provide Only Temporary Relief,* 257 J.A.M.A. 220 (1987).

Another useful way to discuss health care rationing is to identify the social and institutional levels at which it occurs. At the most global level, society can decide how much of its total resources to devote to health care versus other social needs, as the British Parliament does when it sets a budget for its National Health Service. At the most microscopic level, we can focus on which patients receive which treatments, as occurs when decisions are made about who has priority for scarce life-saving organ transplants. At the intermediate level, a rationing analysis can help decide which of the many branches of medicine are over or under-funded. This occurs, for instance, in debates over whether health insurance should cover preventive medicine.

Each of the various cost-containment mechanisms we consider targets one of these levels and then spreads its effects throughout the other levels, resulting in rationing decisions of different forms and content. Before seeing how this happens in more concrete detail, we will explore other dimensions of rationing that are relevant at any of these levels.

2.   The Ethics of Health Care Rationing

The inevitability of health care rationing requires us to confront two difficult questions: what are the criteria for rationing, and who should make the rationing decisions?

a.   Rationing Criteria

The proper criteria for rationing medical care have been debated in a number of contexts. Most prominently, Chapter 6 discusses the criteria used to allocate a limited supply of life-saving organs for transplant. Later in this chapter, we discuss which areas of medical treatment should be covered by public and private insurance. In both discussions, there are common themes that point to contrasting ethical criteria.

One ethical approach is to use "neutral," non-medical criteria that avoid the tough value choices and trade offs. For instance, we could decide which of two candidates should receive an organ transplant by tossing a coin or by picking the one who requested first, but these are usually viewed as arbitrary tie-breakers to be used only when more substantive criteria fail to provide a clear answer.

Which of several substantive criteria should we use? There are two basic approaches: medical need, and medical benefit. The two are not the same, since a patient who is in greatest need may be closest to death and so have the least chance of improving from the treatment in question. Imagine an organ transplant for a desperately ill patient who is likely to die in any event. More medical benefit can be gained by treating someone whose odds of surviving would increase from 50 to 100 percent than by treating someone whose odds would increase from 0 to 20 percent. For this reason, medical researchers have focused considerable efforts on developing objective measures of medical benefit.

One simplistic measure is age. Some ethicists, most notably philosopher Daniel Callahan, argue that health care allocation should favor the young over the old, under the view that this is where it is likely to do the most good. But this rough proxy is not always accurate. Compare a severely deformed newborn infant with a healthy active 70 year old who has a bacterial infection. A more nuanced measure of medical benefit is needed.

Medical benefit could be measured simply by the odds of saving a life, but some people live longer than others, so number of life-years saved is often used instead. But, some people might survive only to live a miserable, painful and disabled existence whereas others might be restored to full health. To account for these possibilities, medical researchers often use a measure of benefit known as a QALY, for quality-adjusted life-year. This is a unit of measure that discounts the number of years added to life by a factor that reflects the degree of diminished quality of life. Thus, one treatment that might produce 10 years of life but with great pain and disability might receive a score of only 5 QALYs, and a different use of the same medical resource that produced 10 years of life in a permanent coma might receive a score of less than 1 QALY.

Making these comparisons is obviously a moral challenge, but if this can be done, then a measurement system would exist that would allow difficult comparisons to be made across not only different patients eligible for the same treatment, but also across different treatments and different diseases. For instance, a public insurance program faced with a difficult budget deficit could decide to allocate limited funds to prenatal care rather than to lifesaving liver transplants if it documented that the prenatal care would produce more QALYs per dollar spent. An example of this approach from Oregon is discussed below.

Although QALYs do a better job than other rationing criteria, there are a number of compelling objections. First, there is no satisfactory way to make the quality adjustment that trades off life for various functional or mental impairments. One could ask people at random how many years of life they would be willing to lose in order to avoid certain conditions, but can we really trust their answers, and who do we ask: only those who have experienced the condition, or only those who haven't? And, what do we do if answers vary widely? Even if these dilemmas could be solved, note that there is a disturbing utilitarian characteristic of QALYs, which is to equate 10 years of life for one person with 1 year of life for 10 people. Most everyone's intuition says the latter is a much greater benefit since more people are saved, but QALYs say the benefits are equal.

b. Rationing Decision Makers

It is certainly possible to fine-tune QALYs or other sophisticated techniques, but we can never expect these tools to resolve all the difficult dilemmas encountered in health care rationing. Ultimately, decisions must be made with imperfect information and unresolved social values and moral theories. How these issues are ultimately resolved therefore depends to a great degree on who the decision maker is. There are, broadly speaking, two alternative mechanisms for making rationing decisions: incentives and rules. Financial incentives, such as those inherent in various forms of prospective payment, can be directed to patients or providers to bring more cost-consciousness to their discretionary decisions. Alternatively, regulatory "command and control" mechanisms can be used to dictate rationing decisions. Both approaches have considerable merit, but they each have serious drawbacks as well.

Directing financial incentives at patients means requiring them to have less comprehensive insurance and to pay more out of pocket. This idea is discussed more below under the topic of medical savings accounts. It certainly has merit, but it faces these fundamental obstacles: Many patients simply cannot afford to pay out of pocket for a significant portion of their care. This is true not just for the poor, but also for those who are elderly or chronically ill, for whom predictable medical expenditures would consume far too much of their income.

For the generally healthy middle class, paying more out of pocket is feasible, but for many is not desirable. Nobel prize-winning economist Kenneth Arrow was the first to expound the "uncertainty" theorem that explains the prevalence of health insurance: Serious disease and accidents are expensive and dreaded events whose occurrence is not predictable; consequently, few people are able to plan rationally for the possible medical expenses simply by setting aside money or absorbing the costs when illness arises. People like comprehensive health insurance because they do not want to agonize over cost/benefit trade-offs when they are anxious about their health or that of a loved one. People generally are also not well informed to make cost/benefit trade-off decisions on their own, so they rely heavily on their physicians' advice. Therefore, it makes more sense to keep insurance comprehensive and direct financial incentives to physicians. They have the strongest influence on medical decisions as well as the best information.

These points are confirmed to some extent by a large-scale social experiment conducted by the RAND Corporation in the late 1970s and early 1980s. These researchers randomly assigned people to different types of insurance. Those assigned to so-called "catastrophic insurance," which required them to pay much more out of pocket, indeed ended up spending considerably less on their health care. But these savings came primarily from decisions not to consult a doctor in the first instance. Once people consulted a doctor, they tended to incur the same costs regardless of how much they paid out of pocket. Also, analysis showed that the initial decisions not to seek care were not well informed. People did not accurately differentiate when they really needed to see a doctor and when then did not. Also, people who started the experiment both poor and sick ended up with measurably worse health status if they had to pay out of pocket, even though the research protocol gave them sufficient funds to pay for the uninsured part of their medical costs.

Financial incentives directed at physicians raises its own concerns, however. An imposing weight of ethical opinion supports the view that doctors should never allow their clinical judgment to be influenced in any manner by cost considerations. These ethicists insist that, because doctors act as fiduciary agents for their patients' welfare, they may not compromise optimal medical outcome in order to save money, especially if their patients are not responsible for any of the incremental costs of treatment decisions. The leading advocate of this view is Robert Veatch in A Theory of Medical Ethics 283–85 (1981). *See also* Charles Fried, Rights and Health Care—Beyond Equity and Efficiency, 293 New Eng.J.Med. 241, 243 (1975) ("The physician who withholds care that is in his power to give because he judges it is wasteful to provide it to a particular person breaks faith with his patient."); Norman Levinsky, The Doctor's Master, 311 New Eng.J.Med. 1573 (1984) ("physicians are required to do everything that they believe may benefit each patient without regard to costs or other societal considerations").

This ethical perspective potentially finds expression in the law through the doctrine of informed consent. If physicians are called upon to make rationing decisions, the courts will be confronted with whether it is a violation of the duty of informed consent to withhold a treatment option that the doctor views as not worth its cost, without informing the patient that this resource constraint is being imposed. It might be objected that the duty of informed consent applies only to potentially harmful decisions to treat, but broader theories of informed consent would appear to cover treatment *refusals* as well. *See* Truman v. Thomas, 165 Cal. Rptr. 308 (1980); Gates v. Jensen, 595 P.2d 919 (Wash.1979). Whether these theories require disclosure of economic costs as well as of medical risks is an open question.

The ethical response is that, following the logic of the principal-agent theory just stated, it is at least ethically permissible, if not essential, for physicians to consider costs if doing so makes insurance more affordable or comprehensive. Patients might prefer their doctors to make the necessary cost/benefit trade-offs, considering that the alternatives are worse. This second-best or least-worst conclusion can be reached by employing hypothetical contract analysis such as that developed by philosopher John Rawls. It can also be reached through actual contracts, if patients choose their insurance fully aware of the role their physicians play in containing costs. This again underscores the merits of disclosing the financial arrangements under which physicians are paid.

Nevertheless, it is still troubling when physicians compromise optimal treatment not only to save money for the patient, but also to benefit themselves. This conflict of interest is in sharp contrast to the situation in England where salaried doctors make rationing decisions within a closed budgetary system. In that case, it can fairly be said that any money saved on one patient goes to help another whom the physician considers to be in greater need. In the United States, under HMO insurance and other forms of prospective payment, physicians or private insurers personally profit when they ration care. It is this conflict of interest that ethicists find most disturbing about provider-directed rationing. Because of it, many ethicists conclude that, if decisions to limit spending are imposed, they should come only from neutral sources external to the doctor-patient relationship, such as expert panels, citizen committees, or political representatives.

However, legislative or administrative regulation, which operates under the glare of the public eye, seems inherently incapable of making and enforcing the difficult decisions required in rationing health care. Regulators frequently capitulate to the intense pressure brought to bear by public and private interest groups. Even when regulators perform faithfully and evenhandedly, they necessarily do so according to a uniform standard, based on their view of the consensus opinion or prevailing values in the body politic. A monolithic response may be inappropriate, however, in a pluralistic society where people have widely varying views of what is best or desirable in a particular case.

3.   The Economics of Health Care Rationing

a.   *Free Markets vs. Government Controls*

Comparing incentives with rules raises not only ethical questions but also issues of economic and political theory. The focus of much of the debate over health care reform is on whether market-based solutions are preferable to government intervention. This theme arises in many different contexts, and few people believe that the debate can be resolved cleanly in favor of one side or the other in any absolute sense. Workable solutions will surely require combinations of both points of view.

Also, it is important to stress that the two opposing approaches are not mutually exclusive. As we discussed above with respect to financing reform, cost containment reforms lie on a spectrum of greater or lesser degrees of government controls versus free markets. For instance, we will see below that government programs can use market-like incentives rather than rules to "regulate" behavior. Similarly, private insurers subject to market forces can adopt internal rules that control physician and patient discretion. Also, markets can be allowed to function under rules and constraints monitored by the government. Rather than advocate one approach over the other, this section describes the themes and characteristics of market versus regulatory approaches in the abstract, to help critique particular reform ideas as they are encountered later.

One such characteristic has already been noted, namely, that markets tend to permit a much broader range of value choices to be expressed than do government systems, which tend to impose a more uniform solution. On the other hand, decisions made in government systems are more visible and therefore more subject to open debate. While this visibility lends to the legitimacy of the resulting decisions, it also makes it more difficult to make tough decisions, and it subjects these decisions to more political pressure by affected interest groups. Government also tends to implement its decisions through coercive, regulatory means, which people resist through evasion, circumvention or outright defiance. Enforcement therefore can be costly and ineffective. In contrast, markets operate through incentives and rewards, thereby achieving their objectives mainly through voluntary action.

These factors appear to point to market solutions as preferable, where they are available, which captures the political morality that prevails in other segments of the American economy. The difficulty is that market approaches may not be viable in health care because of its unique characteristics. The most obvious obstacle to the operation of competitive forces in the health care market is the existence of insurance. The fact that someone else is paying creates what is known as a "moral hazard" problem, meaning that the purchasing decisions of patients and providers are distorted by the presence of insurance.

Second, many people have a fundamental philosophical opposition to pursuing a market-oriented mentality in health care. These critics maintain that such a mentality tends toward excessive commercialization and routinization of what should be a caring, individualized service. They view the hard-edged market as incompatible with the "soft," intangible values that we treasure in the healing arts, and they maintain that competition is incompatible with health care "as a caring rather than purely a curative activity, the goal of which is to reduce pain and anxiety and increase the patient's sense of self-determination and quality of life." Rand Rosenblatt, *Health Care, Markets and Democratic Values,* 34 Vand.L.Rev. 1067 (1981).

Despite such criticisms, competitive forces are increasingly evident throughout the health care sector, as will be seen in the following section. To some extent, competition is focused directly on medical care decisions, with patients paying more out of pocket and with hospitals and drug companies engaging in direct advertising to consumers. For the most part, however, competition is focused at the level of insurance purchase. It is felt that, even if market forces do not work well for discrete items of care, these forces are capable of shaping the structure of insurance, which in turn sends institutional and monetary signals to physicians, hospitals and patients about how medical care decisions should be made. As noted above, even Medicare and Medicaid are turning to market-like voucher systems in which people receive coverage by enrolling with private HMOs.

b. Economic Theory

Even if an explicitly market-based approach is not adopted, still, economic analysis can help us understand what the ultimate objective should be for a successful approach to health care rationing. From an economic perspective, ideally, resources should be devoted to each medical procedure up to the point that their marginal costs equal their marginal benefits,[1] that is, the point where the last dollar spent produces no more or no less than a dollar's worth of additional benefit. A graphic representation may assist in understanding these concepts. (This analysis is adapted from Clark Havighurst and James Blumstein, *Coping With Quality/Cost Trade–Offs in Medical Care*, 70 Nw.U.L.Rev. 6 (1975).) The following figure displays a hypothetical relationship between marginal increases in health care production and health care quality.

1. "Marginal," in this context, means the incremental cost or benefit attributed to each additional unit of service, as opposed to the *aggregate* value for all services combined, or the *average* value per service. For instance, a hospital's marginal cost for treating its first patient is very high—the cost of the entire hospital—but the marginal cost for its second patient is quite low, since the hospital is already built, the nurses employed, etc. Similarly, the marginal benefit to a patient in cardiac arrest of the first few minutes of life saving care is quite high, whereas the marginal benefit of the last few minutes of a two-week hospital stay is negligible.

Marginal Health Benefits and Marginal Financial

Costs of Additonal Units of Medical Care

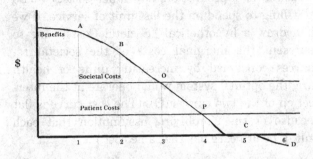

Quantity of Health Care Rendered

The vertical scale is the dollar value of health care (either its benefits or its costs). The horizontal scale represents abstract units of health care (days in hospital, doctor visits, drugs, x-rays, etc.). The "Benefits" curve shows the increment in societal health benefits that result from changes in the quantity of health care provided. Thus, at point A, when little health care is being provided, health care is very productive: there is a large return on each additional resource devoted to medical treatment. At some place down the line, though, we reach a point (B) of diminishing returns where additional health care expenditures rapidly become much less productive. As the line crosses the horizontal axis (point C), we reach the area of totally unproductive care, and below the axis is counterproductive treatment that produces a net medical harm (D).

The marginal benefits curve is in essence a societal demand curve for health care because it tells us, at each level of production, how much society would be willing to spend on the last unit of service. If we then draw a hypothetical "Societal Costs" line to represent the marginal costs of the societal resources consumed by increasing units of health care, the optimal system would operate at the intersection of the two curves (O). (The cost curve is flat because of the simplifying assumption that each unit of health care has the same cost.)

We can also extend this economic analysis to the question of who should be the rationing decisionmaker. The diagram illustrates that where along the benefits curve our system tends to operate depends on the incentives that influence the behavior of the various actors that might make treatment decisions. For instance, under traditional insurance which guarantees providers full payment for any service they render, doctors will tend to function at C, because they seek to derive as much health benefit as possible, regardless of the cost. There is a risk that, if doctors become too focused on the financial rewards, or if they are too concerned about malpractice liability, they may tend to function at D, where providing these additional services leads to an actual decrease in quality of care. Patients may be somewhat more constrained by the payment of coinsurance and deductibles, but if these amount to only 20 percent of actual costs, their cost line will be 80 percent below the level of true societal costs.

We can predict a markedly different outcome under nontraditional reimbursement methods. Criticisms of HMOs and capitation payment suggest they tend to operate near point B because decisions are made by corporate budget cutters who are insufficiently attuned to patients' needs. However, countervailing forces from market competition, malpractice exposure, regulatory oversight, or ethical standards might bring these incentives back in line. The difficulty is that we do not know whether these forces will adequately, excessively, or optimally counterbalance cost-cutting incentives since there is no ideal vantage point from which to measure what is ideal.

Therefore, this sort of analysis cannot generate a precise dollar amount for how much we should spend on any aspect of health care. Nevertheless, it establishes that an optimal health care system avoids spending money not only on unproductive or counterproductive care but also on beneficial care that is nonetheless more costly than it is worth— what might be called marginally unproductive care. One way to evaluate various proposals for containing costs, both regulatory and market-based, is whether they are capable of generating wise decisions about which beneficial treatments are not worth their costs.

D.　COST CONTAINMENT REFORMS

1.　Reducing the Scope of Insurance

a.　Practical Problems

The simplest way to contain costs is to reduce the scope of insurance. This can be done in three different ways: eliminate the bottom layer of coverage by requiring patients to pay entirely out of pocket for most of their routine care. This is known as "catastrophic" insurance, meaning insurance doesn't kick in until medical expenses reach a very high level (say, $3000–$5000) in one year. The second approach is to eliminate the top layer of insurance by capping the total amount that will be paid in any year or over a lifetime. This is called "bare bones" insurance. The third approach doesn't have a common name, but it might be called "swiss cheese" insurance: coverage that is comprehensive for the services included, but which excludes entire categories or service, such as mental health or expensive organ transplants.

There are a number of objections to these approaches. First, they are demonstrably not popular with consumers. Even though economists tell us we have too much insurance, people have a persistent desire to be fully insured, for reasons explained above. Therefore, when these more economical options are made available, they typically sell much less than their sponsors anticipated.

Second, some of these approaches may not save as much money as we might first imagine. Catastrophic insurance, for instance, appears to require that most medical care be paid for out-of-pocket since most people's medical bills never reach the catastrophic threshold in any given year. This is deceptive, however, since most medical spending is concentrated in the small number of people with very high cost illnesses. For these people, catastrophic insurance provides unlimited coverage once they exceed their deductibles.

Even below the deductible level, it is questionable how much out-of-pocket spending will be reduced. The theory is that people will be forced to consider, for instance, whether it is worth it to have a sprained ankle x-rayed for the possibility of a fracture, to visit the doctor for a fever and sore throat, or to undergo an immediate operation for a mild hernia. Some people could not afford any of these options and so would suffer without needed care. To cushion the economic forces, advocates of catastrophic insurance propose to couple them with "medical savings accounts," which are tax-sheltered devices similar to IRAs from which out-of-pocket medical expenses can be paid. But this then begins to look like ordinary insurance, which creates the appearance that someone else is paying. Also, the tax subsidy is expensive.

Another problem with catastrophic insurance is its tendency to aggravate "adverse selection." Catastrophic insurance is much more attractive to the healthy than the sick. Therefore, its lower price reflects not only its greater efficiency, but also the underlying health status of the people who choose it. If catastrophic insurance were to become much more common, the cost of comprehensive insurance might skyrocket as it is left with all the sick people.

Other practical problems limit the potential for bare bones or swiss cheese insurance. Severely limiting the scope of insurance assumes we are willing to deny care to those who choose not to, or are unable to, pay for it. But our society would likely resist the cruelty of denying someone life-saving care because they chose cheap insurance coverage. The "rescue ethic" that prevails in hospital emergency rooms and in intensive care units means that people with limited insurance can free ride on this humanitarian impulse.

b. Disability Discrimination and Other Legal Problems

Cost containment approaches that eliminate entire blocks of insurance coverage also encounter legal obstacles. Under public insurance, these decisions have been challenged as a violation of the statutory mandate to provide all "medically necessary" services or to administer benefits in a nonarbitrary fashion. See Beal v. Doe, 432 U.S. 438 (1977). In a number of cases this medical necessity mandate has proven to be an effective tool for obtaining Medicaid funding of controversial medical procedures. Some courts have gone so far as to require Medicaid to cover medically necessary sex change operations. Rush v. Parham, 625 F.2d 1150 (5th Cir.1980). Most such litigation has focused on decisions by state Medicaid directors to restrict coverage for expensive organ transplants such as livers or hearts. In one decision, the court ruled that Medicaid could not cover liver transplants for some categories of patients but not others, since "to deny services arbitrarily and unreasonably to an otherwise eligible Medicaid recipient in this manner would be impermissible. There are some medical procedures, such as transplants, which Medicaid participation does not obligate the state to provide. However, once these optional services are undertaken, they must be reasonably funded." Ellis v. Patterson, 859 F.2d 52 (8th Cir.1988). In another case, the court required a state to fund a liver transplant for a former alcoholic. Allen v. Mansour, 681 F.Supp. 1232 (E.D.Mich.1986).

Restrictions in the coverage of public insurance have also been challenged as disability discrimination under the American's with Disabilities Act (ADA), and its predecessor, section 504 of the Rehabilitation Act of 1973. 42 U.S.C. § 12101; 29 U.S.C. § 794. The latter applies only to publicly-funded programs and entities, but the former covers private businesses as well. An example of how this law applies to health insurance comes from McGann v. H & H Music Company, 946 F.2d 401 (5th Cir. 1991), which arose prior to the effective date of the ADA. There, the court allowed a private employer to virtually eliminate health insurance for AIDS once it learned that one of its employees was infected with the HIV virus. Now, this is considered to be a clear case of discrimination based on handicap, since HIV infection constitutes a disability, as discussed further in chapter 2. Bragdon v. Abbott, 118 S.Ct. 2196 (1998).

Since virtually any health condition could be classified as a disability, does this mean that health insurance must cover everything in order to avoid disability discrimination? Not necessarily. In Alexander v. Choate, 469 U.S. 287 (1985), the Court ruled under § 504 that a state Medicaid program may cap covered hospitalization at a maximum of 14 days, even though it was clear that this would affect more severely patients who had more serious illnesses and therefore who were disabled. The Court reasoned that the restriction was permissible because it did not specifically target a class of disabled individuals.

These rulings suggest that the cruder and less nuanced is the reduction in insurance, the safer it is under the disability laws. Eliminating entire blocks of service is permissible because this is neutral with respect to disability, but targeting specific illnesses can run afoul of disability discrimination. The difficulty this creates is that, in health policy circles, all efforts are directed at becoming more specific and fine-grained in decisions about what should and should not be covered by insurance. Reductions in coverage like those in Alexander v. Choate constitute "rationing by meat ax," in the words of one commentator (David Eddy), because they eliminate services that might be lifesaving for some patients but allow payment for other conditions where the service might be completely unnecessary. Health policy researchers much prefer to make these cutbacks based on the relative cost effectiveness of the medical service as applied to various medical conditions.

The emerging science of cost-effectiveness evaluation has generated a great deal of controversy. Many ethicists adamantly oppose placing a monetary value on life and health, but cost-effectiveness analysis avoids this by attempting to value alternative methods for incremental medical gains. Without having to decide how much a life or a year of life is worth, it is still possible to evaluate which of several alternative treatments produces the greatest gain, and which does so with the least cost. It is also possible to measure, at the margin, how much incremental gains in life-expectancy cost as advances in medical technology occur. Thus, researchers have calculated that performing a Pap smear every three years to detect cervical cancer costs $12,000 per additional year of life expectancy, but increasing the frequency of testing to once a year costs $930,000 per additional life-year saved. This does not tell us which frequency of testing is correct, but it does help us decide where cuts in funding can be made by doing the least amount of harm, when cuts are necessary.

The most prominent example of using cost-effectiveness techniques for medical technology assessment is the rationing scheme adopted by the state of Oregon to allocate its limited Medicaid funding in a way that allows it to cover all needy people. Most states cover all medical services but are able to afford only about half of people below poverty.

Oregon chose instead to cut back on which services it covered so that it could afford to cover everyone in poverty at whatever level funds allowed. In order to decide how best to cut back on covered services, Oregon created a task force to evaluate the relative effectiveness of the full range of medical services, classified into about 700 categories of conditions and treatments. By eliminating those services that produced the least medical benefit, Oregon was able to afford coverage for only about 590 of these items. This approach was challenged by federal Medicaid administrators as a violation of the ADA, however, because some of the excluded items targeted conditions that constitute classic disabilities, such as liver transplants for alcoholics, and intensive care for severely deformed or premature newborns. Oregon officials had to make extensive revisions in order to salvage their innovative plan.

This solution may appear to work an acceptable compromise between the need to ration scarce medical resources and the concerns over disability discrimination, but in fact it does not. Disability discrimination concerns are still at the core of any effective rationing mechanism even if the most visible categories are avoided. This can be seen best by recalling the discussion above, in section C.2.a, of using "quality-adjusted live years" (QALYs) to gauge the effectiveness of different medical treatments. This measure responds to the concern that mere life expectancy is too crude a measure, since some lives that are saved or lengthened may leave people in severe pain or in a permanent coma. But, adjusting the measure of value according to the quality of life that results from treatment would provide fewer resources to those who end up with greater disabilities. Once again, the more refined and sophisticated are the tools for medical technology assessment, the more likely they are to run afoul of disability discrimination laws. It may be possible to reconcile some uses of QALYs and other cost-effectiveness measures with these laws, but the tension between these two social objectives still lies at the core of rational health planning. The same is true for more covert ways of rationalizing restrictions in treatment, such as the "futility" concept discussed in chapter 7.E.

2. Rigorously Reviewing the Necessity of Care

An alternative to reducing the scope of insurance is to keep insurance comprehensive but to impose a more demanding standard for when services are necessary in particular cases. Most public and private insurance restricts coverage to services that are "medically necessary" and not "experimental." Over the past decade, insurers have become much more demanding about when services are established and appropriate for specific patients or conditions. This has resulted in a spate of litigation concerning the proper interpretation of these coverage terms.

In one line of cases, courts have been very reluctant to allow insurance companies to deny reimbursement based on their determination that the services are not medically necessary. The leading decision is Van Vactor v. Blue Cross Assoc., 365 N.E.2d 638 (Ill.App.1977), where the court reasoned that, because "the term 'medical necessity' is subject to various interpretations, ... there was sufficient evidence to warrant [the trial court's conclusion] that the insured was justified in relying on the good faith judgment of his treating physician" in ordering hospitalization for oral surgery. The court was much more adamant in Mount Sinai Hosp. v. Zorek, 50 Misc.2d 1037, 271 N.Y.S.2d 1012 (1966), which reversed a Blue Cross refusal to pay for three weeks of hospitalization to administer a severe weight reduction diet. The court held that "only the treating physician can determine what the appropriate treatment should be for any given condition. Any other standard would be intolerable second-guessing, with every case calling for a crotchety Doctor Gillespie to peer over the shoulders of a supposedly unseasoned Doctor Kildare."

These holdings have not found uniform acceptance. Other courts have been willing to enforce reimbursement denials, particularly where the insurance policy explicitly states that the insurer has final authority to determine medical necessity. Sarchett v. Blue Shield of Cal., 233 Cal.Rptr. 76, 83 (Cal.1987) ("it is unlikely that any insurer could permit the subscriber free selection of a physician if it were required to accept without question the physician's view of reasonable treatment and good medical practice"); Lockshin v. Blue Cross of Northeast, Ohio, 434 N.E.2d 754, 756 (OhioApp.1980) ("a function, basic to the insurer, is the right ... 'to determine whether ... [a] claim should be allowed or rejected' ").

The outcome of these cases is affected by a number of factors. First, the standard of review is greatly affected by which court the case is in. State courts deciding garden variety contract interpretation cases are much more prone to give the benefit of the doubt to the patient. However, most of these cases are now decided in federal court under a standard of review more lenient to the insurer. This is as a result of ERISA preemption. ERISA is the federal statute discussed in chapter 5.C which preempts certain bodies of state law with regard to insurance that is provided as an employment benefit. Here, the effect of ERISA is to force insurance coverage disputes into federal court, to be decided under principles of federal common law. Following Supreme Court precedent, courts defer to insurers' judgment when the contract declares that insurers have the authority to interpret its terms. Firestone Tire & Rubber Co. v. Bruch, 489 U.S. 101 (1989).

The other change that has affected this area of litigation is the shift from retrospective claims review to prospective utilization review. In the past, coverage disputes arose after treatment was rendered, when claim for payment was submitted to the insurer. Now, insurers require that physicians and patients obtain their advance permission before undertaking an expensive course of treatment. This was intended to avoid the unfairness of refusing to pay after a patient has relied on a physician's advice, but it has created a different hardship. Before, denial of coverage only affected payment, not treatment, but now the effect is to tell the physician not to treat at all. This has brought to the courts very high stakes, life-and-death decisions in which they must decide quickly whether to issue an injunction to order an experimental procedure that might save the patient but which has not yet been clearly proven effective.

The undesirability of resolving medical appropriateness issues in this fashion has prompted a search for superior dispute resolution processes, ones that are quicker and easier to access, that avoid the bias of delegating all authority to insurers, and that bring more expertise to bear than exists in the courts. These issues are likely to be addressed in efforts pending at the time of this writing to enact patient protection legislation for managed care insurance.

This area of litigation has also caused insurers to examine the processes by which they conduct utilization review. Typically, they hire nurses, and sometimes lesser trained staff, to take calls over a toll-free number. Treating physicians or their assistants describe the patients' condition and the proposed treatment, and reviewers compare these indicators with screening criteria the insurer maintains in computerized practice guidelines to determine medical appropriateness. If the computer flags a treatment request as questionable, then the request is reviewed by a physician, often a general practitioner with no special expertise in the medical field in question.

Physicians complain this is a poorly-designed process that nit-picks their professional judgment and dictates patient medical decisions without proper credentials or investigation. They insist that utilization review criteria should be publicly disclosed, and that the personnel should have better credentials. So far, however, regulators and courts have been generally accepting of this process. Regulatory authorities set minimum standards, but so far they have required only that personnel be licensed and that the process provide a quick response. Similarly, in litigation, courts have observed that insurers only purport to make payment decisions, not treatment decisions. Physicians are free to, and perhaps are required to, render care they think is necessary even if they won't be paid. Physicians can also assist patients in appealing coverage decisions they think are wrong. See Wickline v. State, 228 Cal. Rptr. 661 (Cal.App.1986).

Even though detailed utilization review is now a permanent feature of the health care landscape, no one believes that it alone can solve all the tough problems. It is an expensive and clumsy process that reaches only major decisions whose cost warrants special scrutiny. Also, it is limited by the capacity of computerized protocols to capture the complexity and nuance of medical decision making. There are approximately 10,000 medical diagnoses and 10,000 different treatments. Devising thorough and accurate guidelines for each of the billions or trillions of possible combinations based on solid empirical evidence is an impossible undertaking, an insight that is captured in the slogan that medicine is as much art as it is science. Therefore, a broad range of medical practice will necessarily remain subject to individualized professional discretion. To reach this portion of decision making, insurers have adopted a variety of payment innovations that seek to make physicians and hospitals more cost conscious.

3. Reforming Provider Payment

The multitude of payment methods for doctors and hospitals can be better understood if they are arrayed in a spectrum from the most open-ended to the most encompassing. This spectrum looks at the structure of the payment method rather than the absolute amount of payment. At the least restrictive end is fee-for-service payment which reimburses providers for each item of care they deliver. At the most restrictive end is salaried employment for physicians and a fixed, global budget for hospitals, according to which each receives only a single, fixed amount that does not vary in any respect according to the number of services provided. Stretching between these two extremes are various intermediate versions that have greater or lesser aspects of variability or "prospectivity."

In this context, prospective payment means a payment method that fixes the amount of reimbursement in advance of treatment and therefore imposes on the provider some degree of risk or potential for profit. If actual treatment costs are lower than the fixed amount, providers profit, but if more, they absorb the loss. Prospective payment thus attempts to replicate market-like forces by giving providers incentives to economize. Prospective payment can take the form of a fee schedule, in which fee-for-service reimbursement is preserved but the amount per service is fixed by the payor rather than set by the provider. Or, prospective payment can take the more global forms of an annual salary or annual hospital budget. In this section, we will explore the more prominent forms of prospective payment developed by public and private insurers.

a. Medicare Prospective Payment

In 1983, the federal government entirely reformed the traditional Medicare system of retrospective, cost-based reimbursement for hospitals, replacing it with a new "prospective payment system." This provides a good starting point for understanding the complexities of designing an efficient and fair set of payment incentives. First, consider the possible units of service for which hospital payments might be fixed in advance. If Medicare paid hospitals a fixed amount for each day that a patient is hospitalized, hospitals would continue to have an incentive to treat patients as long as possible. If Medicare instead paid hospitals a fixed amount for each Medicare patient admitted, it would undercompensate hospitals that, because of their location or specialization, treat relatively sicker patients and overcompensate community hospitals in suburban locations that cater to relatively healthy patients with comparatively minor ailments. Therefore, the solution Congress chose was to fix an amount for each patient admitted according to the patient's diagnosis.

This diagnosis-based method of reimbursement is known as the "DRG" method of payment—for "diagnosis-related groups." Specifically, Medicare takes all medical diagnoses and groups them according to their relative medical resource consumption. Each of these approximately 480 groups is assigned a weighting factor, which is then used to adjust the average cost of treating all Medicare patients. For instance, the DRG for "all major chest surgeries" carries a weight of about 3.0, reflecting an expensive hospitalization. "Other respiratory surgeries" are placed in one of two groups according to whether they are accompanied by complicating conditions, and these groups are assigned lower weights of about 2.5 and 1.5. With an average cost per case of roughly $7000, the first DRG mentioned pays the hospital $21,000, the second $17,500, and the third $10,500. In each case, this is all the hospital gets, even if the patient has multiple other conditions, but the hospital keeps this entire amount, even if the patient can be treated and discharged much easier and quicker than normal.

The DRG form of prospective payment is not unique to Medicare. It was first implemented in New Jersey as the basis for its regulation of all hospital charges under any form of insurance. DRG payment systems have since been widely adopted by state Medicaid programs and private Blue Cross insurance. They have proved successful in restraining the rate of increase in hospital costs.

Despite this impressive success, few if any health policy analysts are convinced that DRGs will result in lasting reform. First, the DRG system has only limited reach. Initially, it covered only *general, acute-care hospitals.* Excluded were (1) specialty facilities such as psychiatric hospitals, and (2) physicians' fees. The seriousness of these limitations is documented by the one-third increase in Medicare *out*patient expenditures that occurred during the first two years that DRGs applied to *in*patient costs. As a result of this shift in services to more unconstrained reimbursement environments, DRG-type payment methods have been developed for a number of additional facilities, including nursing homes, home health agencies, and hospital-based outpatient services. It is questionable, though, whether DRGs are capable of being extended to the core of medical practice:

paying physicians is far more complicated [than paying hospitals]. When developing a hospital-payment system for Medicare, one must handle 11 million admissions to 7000 hospitals for 475 diagnosis-related groups. Those numbers pale in comparison to Medicare's 350 million claims from 500,000 physicians for 7000 different procedure codes. Moreover, whereas hospitals can average their gains and losses under a prospective payment system across many cases, physicians' smaller caseloads and greater specialization make such averaging much more risky for them. These differences mean that improving the way Medicare pays physicians will be vastly more difficult, both analytically and administratively.

Roper, *Perspectives on Physician–Payment Reform,* 319 New Eng.J.Med. 865 (1988).

Owing to these considerable difficulties, the government appears to have abandoned any attempt to design physician DRGs. Instead, it developed a modified system of fee-for-service reimbursement known as a "relative value scale." The version Medicare developed is known as a "resource-based" relative value scale (RB–RVS for short) because it attempts to achieve some degree of parity in the amount that physicians charge for various services by measuring the relative costs of each service according to the time, mental effort, and technical skill required, as well as differences in the costs of malpractice premiums and specialty training. Such a system does little, however, to alter the existing incentives that continually drive up the volume of physician services.

The ample opportunity that DRGs present for manipulation creates grounds for questioning their effectiveness even within their present ambit. DRGs pay hospitals for each patient admitted; therefore, they carry the potential to induce unnecessary admissions. Even for patients who do need hospitalization, DRGs create an incentive to exaggerate the diagnosis. Hospitals encourage doctors to place their patients in higher-weighted DRGs, a phenomenon known as "DRG creep." Moreover, hospitals attempt to "unbundle" medical treatment so that services are placed in the maximum number of reimbursable categories. For instance, hospitals can receive extra reimbursement by performing diagnostic workups prior to admission and by transferring patients to hospital-owned nursing homes after discharge. This sort of activity is wide-spread, which partly explains why outpatient costs mushroomed at the same time DRGs were introduced.

These abusive practices aside, DRGs may prove ineffective even at their core because of a variety of counteracting incentives and barriers inherent in our health care system. Hospitals may have difficulty responding even in a socially beneficial way to the economizing incentives of prospective payment because hospital costs are almost entirely dependent on the treatment decisions of physicians, who continue to be paid on an inflationary, fee-for-service basis. Legal doctrine detailed elsewhere in this book amply protects doctors from outside, financial influence on their clinical judgment. *See* chapters 5.A (unlicensed and corporate practice of medicine), 5.E (referral fee prohibitions), and 3.B (access to the medical staff). Even if such influence could be brought to bear, malpractice laws and the forces of quality competition might deter any lowering of the intensity of service.

The DRG system has also been subjected to vigorous criticism for its several potentially serious negative consequences. Most serious is an allegation that prospective payment leads to inadequate care. Hospitals have been accused of discharging their patients prematurely out of an excessive concern over profits. There are scattered reports of patients being told they must leave the hospital while they are still sick because their Medicare coverage has "expired."

Of course, a DRG payment does not run out; it is, by definition, payment in full for all required services. Because the system works on an averaging principle, it is expected that some cases will be losers and some winners. But hospitals do have an incentive to discharge patients "quicker and sicker." Of course this may be the very purpose of the system, since it is intended to avoid the unnecessary indulgence in hospital care that was common under cost-based reimbursement, when patients were allowed to remain in the hospital during the full period of recuperation even though much less expensive alternatives such as nursing homes and home care were entirely adequate for them. Under DRGs, though, one needs to guard against the danger that patients will be discharged when such alternative arrangements have not been made or they are inadequate. Therefore, Medicare requires that hospitals advise patients of their rights to protest and appeal in the event they believe that a discharge decision is premature.

Other, more subtle, potential harms inhere in the DRG system's attempt to pay the average cost of treatment for each patient. Although this payment is adjusted according to the patient's diagnosis, each patient is assigned to only a single DRG and receives only a single payment[2] based on the principal diagnosis, regardless of the severity or number of illnesses the patient has. The very broad range of illness severity within each diagnostic category creates a strong incentive for hospitals to admit less seriously ill patients. This may lead to overtly discriminatory admissions practices, the validity of which can be tested under the principles developed in chapter 2. More troubling, though, hospitals may find subtle methods for "case-mix management" that pass any possible legal scrutiny—techniques such as eliminating burn units, emergency rooms, or other services that tend to attract severe cases, or by relocating from low-income, inner city population centers where patients as a group tend to be sicker. Over time, these incentives might further exacerbate the serious problems of access to health care that certain population groups already face.

Other problems of access to health care might result from a general reactionary response to this tightening of the health care belt. Hospitals that previously provided generous amounts of service to the indigent may no longer be inclined to do so since the government has restricted their ability to cross-subsidize such charity care from insured patients. Likewise, hospitals may be less interested in supporting medical education and research. Decreased reimbursement threatens decreased interest

2. An important exception to this statement exists for cases classified as "outliers," patients whose costs of treatment lie far outside the normal range. Hospitals receive an additional payment for outliers; however, this payment covers only a portion of the costs of extended care.

in medical innovation and technological development. Finally, critics accuse DRGs of reinforcing a general trend toward the commercialization of medicine. These phenomena lead us to ask in chapters 2 and 5 whether various legal avenues such as tort law and tax law can or should be used to strengthen the obligation to render charity care.

The DRG system responds to these problems to some degree by varying the basic payment rate according to various additional factors that reflect the type and location of the hospital. For instance, each of these hospital types receive additional increments to compensate for their higher costs or greater social mission: teaching hospitals, hospitals with a disproportionate share of low-income patients, hospitals that face higher wage costs, and rural hospitals that are the only facility in the area. But, each of these refinements adds greater complexity and administrative controls to what initially was thought to be a simple incentive-driven system.

As a result of these many criticisms, it is clear that DRGs do not hold the final solution to the health care cost crisis. Congress is now attempting to implement less administratively-intensive strategies that rely on a system of competing private HMOs and health plans. Whether in fact these systems are simpler, fairer, and more efficient remains to be seen.

b. *Capitation Payment and Hmos*

A different form of prospective payment known as "capitation" has taken hold in the market for private insurance. The most common embodiment of capitation payment is the HMO, which stands for health maintenance organization. Health policy analyst Paul Ellwood is credited with coining this term in 1970 to describe what had previously been known more descriptively as "prepaid group practice." The new term is meant to emphasize the HMO's focus on preventive care. This focus springs from the fact that providers are paid a single amount per patient enrolled ("per head," hence, "capitated") to cover all of the medical needs for a prescribed time, usually a year. The term HMO is meant to emphasize the positive incentive this creates to keep patients healthy rather than the incentives under traditional fee-for-service payment which pay doctors more the sicker their patients are.

Capitation is potentially a powerful force for cost containment because it dramatically reverses the traditional financial incentives created by health insurance. HMOs profit by treating less rather than more. HMOs also bring cost consciousness to bear precisely at the point of the most informed treatment decisionmaking: the attending physician. In essence HMOs combine the treatment function and the insurance function into a single entity, in contrast with "third-party" reimbursement.

Precisely how capitation incentives affect medical judgment is not yet well understood. In part, this is because the precise financial arrangements within HMOs are complex and vary widely. Capitation defines the method of payment to the HMO as an entity, but it might choose to pay its physicians and hospitals in any of a number of other ways, including salary, discounted fee-for-service, and fee-for-service with various penalty or reward systems that encourage economizing. (These are called "withhold pools" because they usually operate by withholding a portion of the contracted payment to either pay out or forfeit at year end based on whether performance goals are met.)

These methods of physician payment tend to correlate with different forms of HMOs. In group or staff model HMOs, doctors practice together in the same setting, whereas individual practice associations ("IPA") and network model HMOs are a looser contractual association of a larger number of doctors who maintain practices in their individual offices. Staff HMOs usually employ their physicians on a salaried basis. IPAs typically compensate their physicians on a discounted fee-for-service basis supplemented with the bonus/penalty arrangements just described. Group and network models employ a variety of physician payment techniques, the most notable of which is capitation. When HMOs make capitation payments to their doctors and hospitals, they shift much of their financial risk directly to the providers that recommend and render the care.

In a typical arrangement, the HMO might keep 20 percent of the capitation payment it receives (to cover sales expenses, administrative overhead, and profit), and then split the remainder between contracting hospitals and physicians. For instance, each primary care physician might receive 40 percent of the capitation payment for each patient for which she is responsible, to cover all physician services and pharmacy costs, including the costs of specialists to whom they refer their patients for more complex problems. The remaining 40 percent might then be set aside in a pool to pay for hospitalization costs authorized by this physician. If there are shortfalls in the hospitalization pool, these might be absorbed by the HMO or partially deducted from the primary care physicians' pay. Alternatively, under an approach known as "global capitation," a large multi-speciality physician group might accept the full 80 percent capitation payment and then further contract "downstream" with hospitals and specialists.

Whatever the precise arrangement, the consequence is that physicians have strong incentives to economize both by promoting health and by minimizing treatment for the sick. HMOs in fact spend much less on hospitalization than do conventional providers. They use inpatient facilities as much as 40 percent less than traditional fee-for-service practitioners without a large accompanying increase in the ambulatory treatment. And, as discussed in chapter 5.B.3, they do so without demonstrable harm to patients and, by some measures, better results. This financial and clinical success has spurred rapid growth in the industry. HMOs now account for over half of all privately insured people and they are becoming much more prominent in Medicaid and Medicare. Many state Medicaid programs have turned, in whole or in part, to HMOs for health care delivery to the poor. And Medicare promotes HMO enrollment as an alternative.

This fundamental shift in the structure of provider reimbursement raises a host of crucial legal and social issues, most of which are explored elsewhere in this book. Here, we focus on the limits to which HMOs can attempt to influence physicians with financial incentives. Capitation creates a serious conflict of interest between the patient's best medical interests and the physician's economic interest. Many ethicists adamantly oppose any form of financial inducement to bedside rationing, that is, any incentive that would cause physicians to compromise optimal care on account of costs. They reason that this would fundamentally compromise physicians' ethical role as devoted patient advocates, would undermine the trust that is essential to successful therapeutic encounters, and would lead to abuse. Other ethicists and commentators respond that, since rationing is inevitable, some rationing decisions are better made through the nuanced, discretionary, and patient-sensitive judgment that is possible only at the bedside. They reason that, if bedside rationing is to occur, some forms of financial motivation are permissible, if not ideal, and the legal response should be regulatory, not prohibitory. See Mark A. Hall, Rationing Health Care at the Bedside, 69 N.Y.U. L. Rev. 693 (1994).

This basic conflict in perspectives underlies many branches of emerging health care law. It influences malpractice law, informed consent obligations, and patients' rights legislation as they affect HMOs.

Here, we will focus on regulatory law that directly
limits these financial incentives or that requires
their disclosure. The primary source of law is a
statute and set of implementing regulations directed to Medicare or Medicaid patients in hospitals and
HMOs. 42 U.S.C. §§ 1320a–7a(b)(1), 1395mm(8)(A);
42 C.F.R. § 417.479. For hospitals, this law takes a
prohibitory approach. It flatly bans any "payment,
directly or indirectly, to a physician as an inducement to reduce or limit services provided with respect to [Medicare or Medicaid patients who] are
under the direct care of the physician."

For HMOs, however, this law takes a more permissive, regulatory approach. It bans only financial
incentives directed to a single patient and that are
designed to limit care that is medically necessary.
Other incentives are allowed, however, according to
various parameters that affect their strength and
immediacy. For instance, financial incentives that
affect only physicians' time and effort and not their
income, such as capitation for primary care physician services, are not restricted. Also exempt from
regulation are incentives that are pooled across a
group of doctors who treat a large number of patients (25,000) so that withholding care for any one
of them does not impose any substantial penalty on
the responsible physician, yet the group has an
incentive to economize on all care. Finally, the
Medicare regulations require certain safeguards,
oversight measures, and "stoploss" protections for
incentive arrangements that put more than 25 percent of a physician's compensation at risk.

This complex regulatory approach, which permits some incentives, bans some, and limits some, is likely to become the legal norm as these rules are adopted by states and applied to private insurers. In addition to whether these incentives are permissible, the law must determine the extent of their disclosure. As discussed in chapter 2.B.3, plaintiffs lawyers are beginning to argue in malpractice litigation that failure to disclose financial arrangements with HMO physicians that create a conflict of interest violates the fiduciary nature of the treatment relationship and constitutes lack of informed consent to treatment. A number of states require by statute that these and other disclosures be made to HMO subscribers.

4. Public Utility Regulation

DRG prospective payment and HMO capitation create passive, market-based reimbursement incentives to control medical costs. In contrast, a much more heavy handed, "command and control" regulatory approach could be employed. This is the approach embodied in the certificate of need laws (CON) enacted in the 1970s (discussed in chapter 3.A.2), which require agency approval before making capital expenditures or offering new services. This approach is also embodied in so-called "all-payor" hospital rate regulation, which a number of states (mostly in the Northeast) instituted in the 1970s and 1980s. All-payor rate regulation takes a prospective payment method such as DRGs or global budgeting and applies it uniformly to all sources of payment, including private insurance and out-of-pocket payment. In essence, hospitals are treated like regulated monopolies, similar to electric companies, local telephone service, and other public utilities.

This approach is currently not in vogue. All-payor rate regulation has proven ineffective, and it has been repealed in almost every state that tried it. The federal requirement for state CON laws has also been repealed. Nevertheless, elements of the public utility approach remain. CON laws still exist in most states, and prospective payment methodologies imposed by Medicare and Medicaid maintain a considerable degree of federal and state rate regulation. Whether the public utility approach will be revived in the future remains to be seen. This is how hospitals are regarded in Canada, England, and other countries with universal health care systems, and it is how many critics allege the Clinton reform plan would have treated health insurers.

E.   RECAPITULATION

Several themes emerge from the policy discussion in this chapter that have central relevance to the doctrinal topics addressed in the following chapters. First, studying the legal infrastructure that buttresses the traditional institutions and relationships in medicine will help us better understand the causes of the crisis in health care spending. Second, in a time of tremendous ferment, experimentation, and change, it is critical to recognize the numerous

challenges this upheaval will present to conventional legal thinking as it struggles to adapt past doctrine to the new circumstances. Third, there is a
mind-boggling array of legislative and market strategies for containing costs and expanding access, and
an equally daunting array of anticipated responses
from insurers, providers, and patients. While it is
helpful in understanding this complex tapestry to
sort reform techniques into market-based versus
regulatory approaches, this does not resolve which
approach is best or is most likely to take hold.
Virtually every reform technique that has been conceived exists in some form or fashion in the highly
fragmented and hugely complex set of institutions,
laws, and policies that make up the American
health care "system."

CHAPTER 2

THE TREATMENT RELATIONSHIP

Any treatment of health care law faces the daunting task of deciding which topics to present and in what order. Health care law, as it has developed over the past four decades, has become an unwieldy collection of disparate areas of doctrine and public policy. Accordingly, some lawyers and scholars maintain there is no unifying structure or core set of ideas that qualifies this as a coherent and integrated body of legal thought and professional practice, other than the happenstance that each topic involves doctors, hospitals, or health insurance in some way. We agree this field has not yet gelled in the way that classic first-year law school subjects have, but we nevertheless see interlaced throughout these disparate topics several organizing principles or themes that potentially explain not only what makes these disparate parts cohere, but also why that coherence distinguishes health care law from other bodies of law.

One of these organizing themes, and perhaps the most prominent, is the set of attributes that make the medical enterprise uniquely important or difficult in the legal domain. Health care law is about the delivery of an extremely important, very expensive, and highly specialized professional service. If anything distinguishes health care law, it must be the unique aspects of the treatment encounter viewed from both sides of the doctor-patient relationship. Health care law in each of its branches must take account of the phenomenology of what it is to be ill, to seek treatment, and to be a healer. These human realities are permanent features that distinguish this field from all other commercial and social enterprises and alter how generic legal doctrine and conventional economic and political theories respond to its issues and problems.

Accordingly, this chapter focuses on the doctor-patient relationship. The first part explores the legal rules that govern the *structure* of the treatment relationship: the duty to treat, and the formation and termination of the relationship. The second part looks more into the *content* of the treatment relationship. It surveys the legal doctrines and policies that flow from the fiduciary nature of the relationship, including confidentiality, informed consent, and the contractual modification of treatment obligations.

A. DUTY TO ACCEPT AND TREAT PATIENTS

The ability (or inability) to pay for medical services strongly affects legal rights of access to care. On the other hand certain obligations to treat are independent of the ability to pay, and, even for paying patients, there remain some barriers to treatment based on race, disability and other factors. Throughout the following discussion, attention is given both to the special problems of access to care by the indigent, and to those general principles governing the duty to treat that apply irrespective of a patient's financial circumstances.

1. Doctors

a. The "No–Duty" Rule

A doctor is generally under no duty to accept patients, regardless of the seriousness of their condition, their ability to pay, or the physician's basis for refusing. In the seminal decision, which is still regarded as stating "good" (*i.e.*, prevailing) law, the court affirmed the dismissal of a suit for damages on behalf of a would-be patient who died when a physician refused to treat her—notwithstanding that the doctor had been her family physician in the past, was available to render care (and aware that other physicians were not), was told she was now seriously ill and relying on an expectation of treatment, gave no reason for the refusal, and was offered payment. Hurley v. Eddingfield, 156 Ind. 416, 59 N.E. 1058 (1901). The court reasoned that a physician's traditional freedom to select patients remained unaltered by the advent of state licensure law, which imposed no obligation on a physician "to practice at all or on other terms than he may choose to accept." In a more recent Texas case, a doctor refused to attend to a pregnant "Negro girl in the emergency room having a 'bloody show' and some 'labor pains' "; as a result, the baby lived only 12 hours. The court had no qualms about pronouncing:

Since it is unquestionably the law that the relationship of physician and patient is dependent upon contract, either express or implied, a physician is not to be held liable for arbitrarily refusing to respond to a call of a person even urgently in need of medical or surgical assistance provided that the relation of physician and patient does not exist at the time the call is made or at the time the person presents himself for treatment.

Childs v. Weis, 440 S.W.2d 104 (Tex.Civ.App.1969).

This "no-duty" rule tracks the historical absence, in American tort law, of any legal obligation to aid strangers in distress. Professional medical ethics reflect a similar policy: "Even the Hippocratic Oath, by which every doctor is morally bound, assumes a pre-existing relationship of patient and physician, which relationship in its inception is basically contractual and wholly voluntary," Agnew v. Parks, 343 P.2d 118, 123 (Cal.App.1959), and the AMA Principles of Medical Ethics leave a physician free "to choose whom to serve" (though they recognize an exception for emergencies).

Implicit in these articulations of the "no duty" rule is the axiom that, where a physician/patient (or hospital/patient) relationship *does* exist, there *is* a legal obligation to treat. This duty to treat is fiduciary in nature (sec. B.1.) and persists until the relationship is properly terminated (sec. A.6). Since the formation of the treatment relationship is foundational to the entire range of issues that make up law and medicine (including malpractice and most of bioethics), what constitutes "formation" is important.

b. Formation of the Treatment Relationship

The court in *Hurley v. Eddingfield, supra* absolved Dr. Eddingfield despite his having been the deceased's "family doctor." This reflects the general rule that an established custom of past treatment does not oblige a doctor to treat a patient's future illnesses; doctor/patient relationships are specific to a "spell of illness" and must be established, or renewed, accordingly.

Within a given "spell," however, the law often requires very slight involvement before finding that a treatment relationship between patient and doctor (or hospital) has been formed. A patient's description of symptoms over the phone followed by a physician's brief instructions, a telephone call to a physician's office for the purpose of initiating treatment, or scheduling an appointment to treat a particular medical problem have all sufficed to support a factfinder's inference that a doctor or hospital had undertaken to provide care. While little is generally required, the decisions are not uniform: courts have also found that no relationship arose where the call to a physician's office to schedule an appointment did not itself seek or generate medical advice, and that where a patient *interpreted* the physician's response to her telephone contact as a refusal to undertake care, the requisite "consensual" characteristic of the relationship was missing—irrespective of the objective content of their communication.

Physicians' informal "curbside" consultations with colleagues normally will not establish a relationship between the patient and the consultee-physician. Reynolds v. Decatur Memorial Hospital, 660 N.E.2d 235 (Ill.App.1996). The *Reynolds* court argued that to imply a treatment relationship out of limited, routine consultative contacts (of which the patient, incidentally, is often unaware) would chill a useful medical practice, to the detriment of patients and physicians alike. Of course, more formal physician referrals likely *will* result in legal recognition of the treatment relationship.

Finally, no treatment relationship customarily arises where physicians examine patients for the benefit of third parties. Thus physicians conducting physical exams for insurance eligibility or for employment-related purposes generally are not held liable to the examinee for failure to treat, or for other medical errors or nondisclosures. Exceptions have arisen, however. In the employment context, courts have implied a *limited* relationship, imposing a duty that extends only to disclosure of any test results that "pose an imminent danger to the examinee's physical or mental well-being," or have implied the relationship where the physician affirmatively undertook treatment or gave advice. See, e.g., Green v. Walker, 910 F.2d 291, 296 (5th Cir.1990). At least one case held that an employer *itself* (in contrast to the examining physician) may be liable to the examinee for negligent failure to disclose a serious medical problem discovered in a pre-employment exam. Dornak v. Lafayette General Hospital, 399 So.2d 168 (La.1981). In contrast, in a recent case a life insurer was found *not* to have a duty to disclose positive HIV test results to a policy applicant. However, the court, seemingly unaware of the "no duty" rule usually applied in such situations, suggested in dictum that if a physician (rather than the company) had been "directly involved," the court might find a duty to disclose such information, based on patients' expectations, professional ethics, and physician expertise in health matters. Deramus v. Jackson Nat. Life Ins. Co., 92 F.3d 274 (5th Cir.1996). Of course, to the extent these policy rationales are persuasive, they undercut the no-duty rule that normally applies in these cases.

2. Hospitals

It is sometimes stated that the "no duty" rule documented above for physicians applies with equal force to hospitals. While this *might* have been true at one time (the older case law seems to say so, but it is not without ambiguity), this general "no duty" rule unquestionably is not the law now. Hospitals and other health care institutions, in contrast with physicians, operate under numerous sources of law (both statutory and court created) that prohibit the arbitrary refusal to admit patients.

Before proceeding to an exploration of those developments, it is important to understand that uninsured patients traditionally have relied on free care rendered by public or private hospitals. Most larger cities maintain a municipal hospital that is obliged to treat all patients regardless of the ability to pay, and many smaller localities make provision for the uninsured by compensating private hospitals for treating the poor. This local largesse is quickly becoming overtaxed, however, even to the extent of threatening the bankruptcy of some counties. Private hospitals have a long tradition of caring for the poor, but their capacity for charity care has been stretched thin by recent reimbursement constraints that eliminate the ample revenues previously received from insured patients. As a consequence of these various social forces, we have witnessed a shocking series of well-publicized incidents in which private hospitals turn desperately ill patients away from their emergency rooms, usually by transferring them to public municipal facilities. This practice of "patient dumping" has led both to litigation over a private hospital's obligation to render emergency care to indigent patients and to a new federal law addressing the practice (sec. A.2.b.). Because of this history and the persistence of access disparities, the following two subsections, while exploring hospital treatment duties generally, have particular importance for access to care by the indigent.

a.   The General Duty to Provide Care

Wilmington General Hospital v. Manlove, 174 A.2d 135 (Del.1961) is the seminal decision that finds in the common law a duty on the part of hospitals to act reasonably in their patient selection decisions. *Manlove* involved a hospital emergency room that refused to treat a severely ill infant because he was under the care of another physician who was not a member of the hospital's medical staff. As a result, the infant died. By analogy to the tort of negligent termination of gratuitous services, the court reasoned that in cases of "unmistakable emergency," a hospital that maintains an emergency room which by "established custom" has been open can properly be held responsible for refusing to treat a patient whose condition "worsens" as a consequence of time lost pursuing the unforthcoming treatment. Detrimental reliance is thus at the core of the case. Accordingly, *Manlove* applies only to emergency care, and even then its scope is rather limited. (Section A.2.b.1, *infra*).

A potentially more powerful and sweeping common law theory—one that would cover *all* forms of hospital treatment—asserts that private hospitals owe duties to the public at large on the ground that they are "quasi-public," by virtue of the importance of their services, the funding they receive from public sources, their licensure, and their tendency to enjoy monopoly status in a community. Chapter 3.B.4 explores in some detail the notion, accepted in some states, that such "quasi-public" status has importance in the context of *physicians* seeking access to a hospital; it is even more to the point with respect to *patient* access. The *Manlove* court rejected this view, however, and it has not in fact been widely adopted, although a few courts have been receptive to it. See, e.g., Leach v. Drummond

Med. Group, 192 Cal.Rptr. 650 (Cal.App.1983) (reasoning applied to the only physician group practice in town).

b. Access to Emergency Care

Notwithstanding the absence of a general duty to rescue, in certain areas the law has been slowly (perhaps even ambivalently) but perceptibly responsive to the moral challenge of taking action to reduce acute, visible and avoidable suffering. One of the areas in which this trend may be at work is in the legal recognition of a hospital duty to care for emergency patients irrespective of their ability to pay.

(1) Common Law and Statutory Rights

Manlove was the first case to fashion a theory of relief for patients denied hospital emergency care. Its principal impact has been in securing access to emergency care by uninsured patients. In addition, about half the states have laws expressly requiring hospitals to treat emergency patients without regard to their ability to pay. Federal law imposes the same duty on hospitals that have received federal assistance under the Hill–Burton Act (42 C.F.R. § 124.603(a),(b)), although these requirements have not been systematically enforced, and on those hospitals that maintain charitable tax exemption (discussed in chapter 5.D).

These established legal protections are limited, though, by their narrow definitions of what constitutes an emergency and of the extent of treatment required in an emergency. For instance, the *Manlove* theory, applied in a number of states, addresses refusals to treat only in cases of "unmistakable" emergency, only where the patient's condition worsens due to the delay in finding an alternative source of care, and only where the delay is caused by reliance on an ER's open-door custom. Many of the state statutes define an emergency as a situation requiring immediate treatment in order to prevent loss of life or limb—which can exclude a broad range of serious, albeit less extreme, medical conditions.

Two Arizona cases point the way toward a more expansive duty to provide emergency care. Eschewing *Manlove*'s reliance-based approach, the Arizona Supreme Court has implied a sweeping duty "to provide emergency care to *all* persons presenting themselves for such aid" (emph. in original), ostensibly based upon the state regulatory requirement that all general hospitals maintain emergency facilities as a condition of licensure. Guerrero v. Copper Queen Hospital, 537 P.2d 1329 (Ariz.1975). A decade later the court relied on JCAHO standards prohibiting discrimination based on the "source of payment," incorporated by reference into the state's hospital licensing statute, to conclude that hospitals may never transfer emergency patients for economic reasons. Thompson v. Sun City Community Hospital, 688 P.2d 605 (Ariz.1984).

Guerrero and *Thompson* are important for two reasons. First, they are best understood as based in

common law public policy—essentially, an emergency room application of the "quasi-public status"
theory discussed above—rather than on idiosyncra-
sies of state regulatory law, and are thus of general
rather than parochial interest. Second, they allow
courts to redefine the nature of an emergency and
the extent of the treatment required. Hospitals are
obliged to treat any patient with a "need for immediate attention" and to provide such patients all
care that is "medically indicated." The duty to treat
thus encompasses far more than care necessary to
prevent the patient's condition from deteriorating:
"The relevant inquir[y] ... d[oes] not relate to
'stabilization' and 'transferability,' but rather to the
nature and duration of the emergency." 688 P.2d at
611. This broadened theory has not as yet been
adopted by other states, perhaps due to the subsequent enactment of, and widespread reliance on,
EMTALA—notwithstanding EMTALA's own argua-
ble limitations in this connection.

(2) The Emergency Medical Treatment and Active Labor Act

The Emergency Medical Treatment and Active
Labor Act ("EMTALA"), 42 U.S.C. § 1395dd, was
originally enacted as part of the Consolidated Omni-
bus Reconciliation Act of 1985 ("COBRA"). In recent years this federal law has become the single
most important legal tool governing access to emergency care, due principally to its uniform national
applicability and its remedies. Hospitals that receive

Medicare payment must comply with EMTALA's terms for *all* their patients. EMTALA creates a private right of action for damages for violation of its terms by such hospitals, though there is no comparable action against physicians. It also authorizes civil money penalties up to $50,000 for negligent noncompliance by both hospitals *and* physicians.

EMTALA was enacted in the belief that state law was too weak to prevent the widespread "dumping" of indigent and uninsured patients. Its protections, however, go further: they are triggered by the refusal to properly examine or treat "any individual" who comes to a hospital emergency department seeking care, irrespective of the person's eligibility for Medicare or whether he can pay for care. Brooker v. Desert Hospital Corp., 947 F.2d 412, 415 (9th Cir.1991). EMTALA requires, first, that the hospital provide for an "appropriate medical screening examination within the capability of the hospital's emergency department," to determine whether there is a medical emergency. If so, treatment must then be provided to the point of "stabilization." Specific analogous provisions also apply to women in labor.

(a) Screening

A moment's reflection on the statutory language just quoted suggests that a diagnostic screening might be "[in]appropriate" in varying ways, and for different reasons. Uncertainty has thus arisen over just what hospital conduct the statutory phrase reaches, as well as what standard of performance it imposes.

Many courts assert that the essence of an EMTA-LA screening violation is proof that the patient was harmed by "disparate" or "non-uniform" treatment—some *variation* from the medical practices that the hospital would otherwise apply to similarly-situated persons. This approach focuses solely on whether a hospital complied with its own standard procedures, and many cases have rejected EMTALA claims on the basis that there was no such showing. A variant approach seems to require the existence of an improper *motive* for the disparate treatment, based on factors such as race, sex, ethnic group, politics, or personal characteristics. This has been criticized on the grounds that there is no statutory support for such a reading, that it is so inclusive as to be virtually without limit (and therefore meaning), and that it is nonetheless sufficiently difficult to prove that it would defeat virtually all EMTALA claims. Power v. Arlington Hosp. Ass'n, 42 F.3d 851, 857–58 (4th Cir.1994).

Courts have adopted the "disparate treatment" analysis largely in an effort to avoid making EMTA-LA a federal malpractice law that would displace ordinary state-law negligence claims, a result which they believe Congress did not intend. Vickers v. Nash. General Hosp., 78 F.3d 139, 142–43 (4th Cir.1996) (reviewing cases). However, a type of malpractice law seems inevitably to arise from the judicial requirement of uniform treatment. Uniformity presupposes the hospital has a standard practice against which to measure the alleged variation, and indeed this is often true. Hospitals are compelled by many forces—state licensure laws, their own governing boards and by-laws, JCAHO standards, the threat of malpractice liability—to adopt policies and procedures that are normative, likely embracing accepted standards of professional competence by institutions of comparable size, nature and circumstances, rather than merely allowing idiosyncratic and perhaps sub-standard conditions or practices to take hold unheeded. This is the stuff of malpractice law.[1] Courts will not likely accept a hospital's defense that it *has* no standards against which divergence could be measured, for to do so would encourage such conduct; instead they will impose the relevant tort-law standard of care on the institution. Power v. Arlington Hospital Ass'n., 42 F.3d 851, 858 (4th Cir. 1994). Thus in purporting to require only "equal" or *consistent* care by a given hospital, the disparate treatment test actually imposes a substantive requirement of *nonnegligent* care.

Where an institution deviates from its (nonnegligent) standards through medical error or omission, many courts nevertheless refuse to apply EMTALA, out of a continuing reluctance to federalize all

1. A malpractice-type standard, in fact, is not inconsistent with EMTALA's statutory language for "appropriate" screening "within the capability" of the institution. The former reflects malpractice law's normative, objective content; the latter reflects its recognition that the standard of care may vary with a hospital's treatment category and, perhaps, available resources.

emergency room tort law. Instead, they require a purposeful deviation. Thus where a physician failed to detect chest sounds indicating a broken sternum and rib which would normally prompt a diagnostic X-ray, the court ruled that the failure to X-ray was simple negligence and *not* "disparate treatment" sufficient to state an EMTALA claim. Summers v. Baptist Medical Center Arkadelphia, 91 F.3d 1132 (8th Cir.1996) (*en banc*); accord, *Vickers, supra.* Compare this approach to the *Power* case, where the court characterized the hospital's failure to give the plaintiff a diagnostic blood test—the allegedly negligent error *itself*—as "disparate treatment" sufficient to constitute an EMTALA claim. Although the *Power* court struggled to sustain a formal distinction between EMTALA and malpractice law by observing that only negligent *omission* of a diagnostic test and not negligent *interpretation* or *performance* would support claims under both theories, this decision virtually conflates EMTALA and medical negligence in all cases of omitted emergency treatment.

(b) Treatment and Stabilization.

If the required screening reveals an "emergency medical condition," the hospital must undertake treatment. EMTALA's definition of "emergency" is a condition reasonably likely, without "immediate" treatment, to create "serious jeopardy" to the person's health. This definition is at least as inclusive as many of those found in state common law and state statutes, and the range of conditions it covers is thus reasonably broad.

The more problematic issue is how far treatment must proceed under the statutory mandate to "stabilize" the condition. Stabilization is defined as a level of treatment likely to prevent "material deterioration" of the condition during transfer. (Transfers of *un*stabilized patients are permitted in limited, specified circumstances involving a written request or expected medical benefit). The facts of a pre-EMTALA case, Joyner v. Alton Ochsner Medical Foundation, 230 So.2d 913 (La.App.1970), are instructive. An auto accident victim came to the emergency room of a private hospital with "multiple deep facial lacerations, a possible head injury, traumatic damage to the teeth and multiple bruises and contusions of the body, resulting in considerable loss of blood." The hospital merely bandaged him, took x-rays, monitored for shock and administered I.V. fluids to stabilize his blood pressure before transferring him to a Veteran's Administration hospital for further treatment. This course of action is probably entirely consistent with EMTALA; thus in many situations, EMTALA actually may not require more extensive care than was due under state common and statutory law. Ironically, the expansive treatment obligations in a few common law precedents (see *Guerrero* and *Sun City*, *supra*) may actually *exceed* the "stabilization" requirement of EMTALA. Given EMTALA's dominance of the field, however, their further application seems unlikely, even though EMTALA does not actually preempt such common law claims.

Finally, courts have generally recognized that EMTALA's treatment and stabilization requirement reaches "post-admission dumping" of patients, and thus is not limited to care provided in the hospital's emergency room. Smith v. Richmond Memorial Hosp., 416 S.E.2d 689 (Va.1992). One court, however, refused to apply the stabilization requirement to inpatient care on the ground that it was meant to apply only to the "immediate aftermath" of an encounter for emergency treatment. Bryan v. Rectors and Visitors of the University of Virginia, 95 F.3d 349, 352 (4th Cir.1996).

(c) "Preventive" Dumping

EMTALA requires screening and stabilization of anyone who "comes to" an emergency department. Under this language courts have rejected EMTALA claims by patients who do not, literally, show up at the hospital. E.g., Johnson v. University of Chicago Hospitals, 982 F.2d 230 (7th Cir.1992) (dismissing EMTALA claim where hospital telemetry staff directed paramedics treating child in full cardiac arrest to another hospital). Accord, Miller v. Medical Center of Southwest Louisiana, 22 F.3d 626 (5th Cir.1994) (patient did not "come to" a hospital that refused, by telephone, to take him as a transfer on economic grounds). By regulation, the Secretary of Health and Human Services has confirmed that "comes to" requires physical presence on hospital property; however, a hospital's own ambulance is *deemed* hospital property, and, arguably, non-hospital ambulances cannot be re-routed except for reasons of lack of hospital capacity or staff. 42 C.F.R. sec. 489.24(b).

EMTALA remains controversial. It has been criticized for responding to a problem that was never as widespread as claimed or that no longer exists, and for imposing an awkward and poorly drafted solution. Others believe that EMTALA has been effective; still others that patient dumping persists at unacceptable levels, notwithstanding EMTALA. Under any view, however, EMTALA has become central to the law of access to emergency medical care, and there is little reason to believe its role will decline.

3. Doctors Within Health Care Organizations

How can hospitals, dependent on doctors to deliver care, comply with their institutional duty to treat (under the various legal theories explored above) if *Hurley* leaves physicians free to refuse patients? One solution is regulatory: since EMTALA was enacted, physicians are no longer completely free to refuse emergency patients with impunity, because they may face civil fines for negligent noncompliance with EMTALA's terms. A second solution (pre-EMTALA) is contractual, provided by Hiser v. Randolph, 617 P.2d 774 (Ariz.App.1980). Hospitals may require as a condition of medical staff membership that physicians assist in treating emergency and indigent patients. If physicians accept this condition by joining the medical staff or working in the emergency room, then this contractual obligation may extend to the patient as a third-party beneficiary.

A similar solution applies to managed care, where a health plan may contractually bind participating physicians to see individuals it has a contractual duty to treat. In Hand v. Tavera, 864 S.W.2d 678 (Tex.App.1993), the court relied on the applicable contracts (characteristic of health plans) to find a treatment relationship with an on-call plan physician. The physician refused to authorize the patient's admission to the plan's hospital based on the symptoms and history conveyed by a telephone consult from the ER. As a consequence, the patient had a stroke at home. The court reasoned that the enrollee paid premiums to the plan to purchase medical care in advance of need; the plan arranged to meet its obligation to provide care by paying physicians; those physicians, in return, agreed to treat the plan's members. The *identity* of the physician who happened to be on call for emergency admissions was immaterial: the plan brought the patient and physician together "just as surely as though they had met directly and entered the physician-patient relationship." 864 S.W.2d at 679.

4. Wrongful Denials: Antidiscrimination Law and Refusal to Treat

As discussed thus far, physicians (and, to a considerably lesser extent, hospitals) enjoy substantial legal discretion to refuse patients for "good" reasons, "bad" reasons, or no stated reason at all. In a limited number of areas, which are the subject of this section, federal law specifically disapproves certain bases for treatment refusals. In addition, states often have counterpart regulatory laws, generally applicable to "public accommodations" (which covers hospitals but often not medical offices). The JCAHO's accreditation standards also prohibit discriminatory practices by hospitals on the basis of race and other characteristics, including source of payment, and the federal charitable tax exemption for hospitals carries with it certain obligations to provide care on a nondiscriminatory basis to paying patients.

a. Title VI: Race and Ethnicity

Title VI of the federal civil rights law, enacted in 1964, prohibits any "program or activity receiving federal financial assistance" from discriminating against, excluding, or denying benefits to individuals on the grounds of race, color, or national origin. 42 U.S.C. § 2000d. Thus, overt discrimination by health care institutions participating in the federal Medicare or Medicaid programs (which were enacted in 1965) or receiving other financial support is barred. Despite Title VI, subtler forms of racial (as well as gender) discrimination by health care providers doubtless persist. Title VI has been invoked in a few cases challenging decisions to relocate or to close hospitals serving predominantly minority populations. There is, however, virtually no law exploring the application of the prohibition to physicians.

b. Hill–Burton Obligations

One part of the Hill–Burton law, which provided grant support for hospital construction across the country in the decades following World War II, imposes a requirement that recipient institutions make themselves "available to all persons" in their area. 42 U.S.C. § 291c(e)(1). The regulations implementing this "community service" provision prohibit discrimination against paying patients on the grounds of race, color, national origin, creed, "or any other ground unrelated to an individual's need for the service"; they also disapprove admissions policies that have the "effect" of such discrimination, and require hospitals to ensure access to Medicaid and Medicare patients. 42 C.F.R. s. 124.603(a),(c),(d). Despite their apparent strength, there has been little effort to enforce these obligations. *See generally* Kenneth R. Wing, *The Community Service Obligations of Hill–Burton Health Facilities*, 23 B.C. L. Rev. 577 (1982).

c. Disability Discrimination

Two closely related laws, both of which apply to a wide range of activities beyond health care, are of rapidly growing importance in this field: Section 504 of the Rehabilitation Act of 1973 (29 U.S.C. § 794), and the Americans with Disabilities Act of 1990 (42 USC §§ 12101–12213). HIV/AIDS first drew attention to the application of disability law to health care and HIV cases continue to arise and receive coverage, but the application of disability discrimination law to health care is considerably broader.

The most obvious difference between the two laws is the reach of their regulation. Section 504 applies to *federally funded* "programs and activities" (which includes hospitals that receive Medicare reimbursement, but probably not doctors). The ADA, by contrast, reaches various entities irrespective of whether they receive federal financial assistance, including state and local governments (Title II) and public accommodations (Title III). Of greatest importance here, the latter include the "professional office of a health care provider, hospital, or other service establishment," so doctors' offices are covered. While there is more case law developed under sec. 504 because it has been in effect for so much longer, the greater reach of the ADA suggests that it will ultimately supersede sec. 504 in importance.

(1) Protected Class

The first question in most disability discrimination cases is whether the individual falls within the protected class. Section 504 protects a "handicapped individual," defined as someone with a "physical or mental impairment which substantially limits one or more of such person's major life activities," or someone with either a "record of," or who is "regarded as having," such an impairment. The ADA's definition of "disability", except for the choice of the operative word, is almost verbatim. 42 U.S.C. § 12102(2).

These terms are quite broad, reflecting Congress' intent to protect people against discrimination arising not only from prejudice but also from fear and myth. School Bd. of Nassau County v. Arline, 480 U.S. 273, 279, 284 (1987). Echoing those policies, the Supreme Court recently held that non-symptomatic HIV infection constitutes a disability under the ADA. Bragdon v. Abbott, 118 S.Ct. 2196 (1998).

In *Bragdon* an HIV-positive patient alleged that her dentist violated the ADA when he refused to drill a cavity for her in his office (offering, instead, to do so at a hospital, though there was no evidence the hospital would be safer or even that he had privileges to practice there). The Court held that non-symptomatic HIV infection constitutes (in the statutory terms) a "physical impairment" from the moment of infection onward, and that, by interfering with the plaintiff's reproductive capacity, the infection "affected a major life activity" because of the centrality to life of reproduction and sexual relations. The open-ended nature of this "major life activity" category is suggested by the Court's intimation that other plaintiffs might persuasively assert that HIV impacts *other* life activities, as well. Finally, the Court concluded that HIV infection was a "substantial limit" on the plaintiff's reproductive activity, noting that her status would impose significant risks of infection on male sexual partners (20–25%), and on any child during gestation and childbirth (8%–25%). The Court emphasized that this third requirement is met "even if the difficulties [generated by the disability for the life activity in question] are not insurmountable."

Bragdon not only confirms a decade of consistent judicial and administrative consensus on the specific status of HIV-positivity under § 504 and the ADA, but also, at least equally importantly, bolsters the broad construction of "disability" that the statutory language suggests. For example, the recognition that reproduction is a "major life activity" suggests that a health insurer's exclusion of infertility treatments might be challenged as disability discrimination.

(2) Core Provisions

Finding a handicap or disability is only the first inquiry. Section 504 prohibits regulated programs or activities from excluding, denying benefits to, or discriminating against any "otherwise qualified handicapped individual ... solely by reason of his handicap." 29 U.S.C. § 794. "Otherwise qualified" means able to meet program requirements " 'in spite of' " the handicap, as established through an individualized, factually-specific inquiry. Even where a person cannot initially meet all program or activity requirements, he or she may nonetheless be "otherwise qualified" if the sponsor of the program or activity can make "reasonable accommodation"—i.e., take steps, short of incurring " 'undue financial and administrative burdens' " or making " 'a fundamental alteration in the nature of the program' " (*Arline*, supra), that would enable the person to meet the requirements, in which case the sponsor must do so. The ADA rules, though not identical, are similar. One commentator has concisely summarized the operative core of the two laws:

The superficially distinct requirements that challenged conduct both disfavor a "qualified" disabled applicant and also result in discrimination "on the basis of" disability typically collapse into a single inquiry. As the U.S. Supreme Court observed in *Alexander v. Choate*, [469 U.S. 287, 299 n. 19 (1985)], "the question of who is 'otherwise qualified' and what constitutes improper 'discrimination' ... [are] two sides of a single coin." A person who lacks legitimate qualifications has not been impermissibly discriminated against. Under both statutes, a person is "qualified" to receive services such as health care if, with reasonable modifications, she is able to meet a program's "essential" or "necessary" eligibility requirements.

Philip G. Peters, Jr., Health Care Rationing and Disability Rights, 70 Ind. L. J. 491, 507 (1995).

A key difficulty in disability law is determining whether a person is "otherwise qualified" for the benefit or service. Classical applications of this standard arise in cases involving access to education and employment, in which the analysis has two salient characteristics: (1) it impliedly assumes that the benefit or service is generally available to a qualified class of people, under terms established by its sponsor; and (2) because the disability is not the *reason* for which the person seeks the benefit or service, it is coherent to ask whether the person can meet the eligibility terms *notwithstanding* (or "in spite of") his disability, with any needed reasonable accommodation.

In health care, this analysis applies logically enough where an individual is seeking access to care for a problem that is *un*related to his disability, as where a physician who is treating a patient for an ear infection refuses to perform medically indicated surgery after he learns the patient is HIV positive. Glanz v. Vernick, 756 F. Supp. 632 (D.Mass.1991). The benefit (ear surgery) is generally available on certain terms to those who need it; and, since the patient is seeking care for a condition other than his disability (HIV status), it is coherent to ask whether, with reasonable accommodation (here, relating to his infectiousness and his immunocompromise), he qualifies for the benefit "in spite of" that disability.

But in cases in which it is precisely the disability that *gives rise to* the need for access to health care, this is not a very coherent approach to "otherwise qualified." In Wagner v. Fair Acres Geriatric Center, 49 F.3d 1002 (3d Cir.1995), for example, a nursing home with many Alzheimer's patients denied admission to an agitated, violent 65–year Alzheimer's patient on the ground that the home was inadequately staffed to care for such patients. If one takes at face value the service the home *actually* offered (care for *non-violent* Alzheimer's patients), then the service that the plaintiff *sought* (care for *violent* patients) was simply not one that the home made generally available to a qualified class; viewed this way, the first element of the usual "otherwise qualified" analysis could not be met. It was only by judicially redefining the eligible class—determining that violent patients *should* be admissible to the home (a conclusion buttressed by evidence that the plaintiff could, in fact, be accommodated without unreasonable burden on the home)—that the court could uphold the jury's finding that the plaintiff was "otherwise qualified." Observe, though, that under this expanded view of eligibility, the *second* element of the traditional analysis now becomes incoherent: it makes no sense to ask, " 'In spite of' the fact that she has Alzheimer's disease, is a person eligible for care at a nursing home that takes Alzheimer's patients of all kinds?"

A few courts have found a more meaningful approach in these cases. They preclude a health care provider from using disability *alone* as the basis for withholding medical benefits. A person is "otherwise qualified" for a particular medical benefit if "there is no factor [other than a bona fide medical reason] apart from the mere existence of disability that renders the participant unqualified for the benefit." Woolfolk v. Duncan, 872 F. Supp. 1381, 1389–90 (E.D.Pa.1995) (seeking care for, and alleging discrimination based on, HIV status). For thoughtful commentary on this unsettled problem, see Mary A. Crossley, Of Diagnoses and Discrimination: Discriminatory Non–Treatment of Infants with HIV Infection, 93 Colum. L. Rev. 1581, 1645–54 (1993).

5.   Other Bases for a Duty to Treat

a.   *Constitutional Rights of Access*

It is clear that there is no federal constitutional obligation for government to *fund* health care. The cases involving abortion funding have firmly established that "the Constitution imposes no obligation on the States to pay . . . any of the medical expenses of indigents." Maher v. Roe, 432 U.S. 464, 469 (1977). The due process clause traditionally has been seen as protecting individuals *from* improper government interference ("negative" liberties), rather than generating entitlements *to* state-conferred assistance or benefits ("positive" liberties). E.g., Wideman v. Shallowford Community Hospital, 826 F.2d 1030 (11th Cir.1987). *See also* DeShaney v. Winnebago County Department of Social Services, 489 U.S. 189 (echoing the foregoing).

Violations of negative liberties might be asserted in many contexts of health care regulation. One court found a generalized constitutional right to be free of poorly justified state restrictions on medical decisionmaking. Andrews v. Ballard, 498 F.Supp. 1038 (S.D.Tex.1980) struck down a law that allowed only licensed physicians to practice acupuncture as an infringement of patients' right to "obtain or reject medical treatment," which the court found was encompassed by the right to privacy identified in *Roe v. Wade*. Most courts, however, require only a rational justification and, in any case, they view protecting health as a compelling state interest, so these types of argument rarely succeed. For instance, courts have upheld state bans on alternative cancer therapy that is probably harmless but thought to be ineffective. People v. Privitera, 591 P.2d 919 (Cal.1979). *Cf.* United States v. Rutherford, 442 U.S. 544 (1979).

Even though there is no general constitutional right to health care (as there is in some European countries), "when a State does decide to alleviate some of the hardships of poverty by providing medical care, the manner in which it dispenses benefits is subject to constitutional limitations" imposed by the due process and equal protection clauses. *Maher, supra,* 432 U.S. at 470. Thus, a publicly-funded hospital cannot arbitrarily discriminate in the patients it treats or in the services it provides. *See* Memorial Hospital v. Maricopa County, 415 U.S. 250 (1974) (unconstitutional to refuse county health services to temporary residents).

Another exception to the principle that only "negative liberties" generally enjoy constitutional protection arises when the state has "control" over an individual. Notable litigation has arisen over the treatment rights of institutionalized persons, particularly the mentally ill. The federal courts have held that it is unconstitutional to confine patients involuntarily for the purpose of treatment and then provide no treatment. O'Connor v. Donaldson, 422 U.S. 563 (1975). The most remarkable instance is Judge Frank Johnson's much discussed action taking direct charge of the administration of Alabama's state medical hospital because of its persistent failure to provide any meaningful form of treatment.

Wyatt v. Stickney, 325 F.Supp. 781 (M.D.Ala.1971); 344 F.Supp. 373 (M.D.Ala.1972). Prisoners also gain certain rights to health care by virtue of their confinement, under the 8th Amendment's prohibition of cruel and unusual punishment. See Estelle v. Gamble, 429 U.S. 97 (1976).

b. Patients' Rights

A final source of patients' access rights are so-called Patients' Bills of Rights. In order to comply with JCAHO accreditation standards, hospitals must adopt statements that cover a variety matters related to patient care, including access to care and patient dignity and confidentiality. Although these statements are issued voluntarily, courts probably would give them binding legal force as forming part of the hospital's contractual relationship with its patients. Moreover, in some states these statements are not voluntary. Minnesota is one among several jurisdictions that specify a mandatory bill of rights. On the federal level, a detailed set of protections applies to patients in nursing homes that receive Medicare (42 U.S.C. § 1395i–3) or Medicaid (42 U.S.C. § 1396r) funding.

The rapid growth of managed care in recent years has been accompanied by concerns that health plans are restricting subscribers' access to care by a variety of mechanisms including limiting referrals, restricting coverage, and forcing physicians to withhold information about treatments not offered or covered by the plan (so-called "gag" clauses). As a consequence there has been significant state legislative activity proposing, and in some cases enacting, new patient rights of access. These laws typically require a broader choice of physicians, provide mechanisms to appeal negative coverage decisions and prohibit restrictions on physician communication with patients. As of this writing similar patients' rights legislation is being considered, in several forms, at the federal level.

6. Terminating the Treatment Relationship

We began this chapter with the observation that professional duties arise upon the formation of a treatment relationship and continue until it is properly terminated. Patient "abandonment" is the term applied to an improper termination of treatment that is *intentional*, in contrast with termination that is due to a mistake in medical judgment. The latter is a matter for ordinary malpractice law, but this distinction is frequently confused.

Where a treatment relationship exists, the law of abandonment requires that the physician (or hospital) provide all necessary care unless the relationship is terminated (1) by the patient or (2) by the provider, after giving the patient proper notice and an opportunity to secure an alternate source of care. Abandonment law is thus much more forgiving than is usually recognized. The only explicit restraint on a doctor's (or hospital's) freedom to abandon a patient is the *procedural* one of notice. As classically conceived, there is no real *substantive* content to abandonment law because the law does not scrutinize the *reasons* for abandonment: so far as abandonment law is concerned, a doctor may, with proper notice, stop treatment because he wants to retire, or go on vacation, or simply because he dislikes the patient.

To ensure that there is no question about the adequacy of notice to the patient and opportunity to obtain substitute care, prudent physicians as a practice usually take affirmative steps themselves to arrange for substitute care. A vacationing doctor will usually have an associate cover her cases and a retiring doctor will ordinarily tell patients that a designated physician has agreed to take her cases. Prudent hospitals, likewise, will never simply discharge an ill patient, even after ample notice; instead, they will locate an alternative facility to which a patient can be transferred.

These pragmatic accommodations have created a degree of uncertainty in abandonment law. Because this body of law is based on an implied contractual undertaking and on notions of fiduciary responsibility, its precise limits are not firmly set. Consequently, the case law in different states offers conflicting indications of whether simple notice of treatment termination is sufficient, or whether instead the law requires health care providers to arrange for a substitute source of care.

This point becomes a critical issue in the modern context where doctors and hospitals face increasingly severe constraints in health care reimbursement. A provider might seek to terminate care because the patient's insurance runs out or won't cover the treatment. If patients are given "notice," and perhaps appeal rights, will this suffice under the usual procedural requirements of abandonment doctrine—or might a creative and sympathetic plaintiff persuade a court to read a substantive element into the doctrine, and prohibit the termination of treatment based on inability to pay?

Three cases shed conflicting but ambiguous light on the legality of "economic abandonment." In Ricks v. Budge, 64 P.2d 208 (Utah 1937), the court allowed the plaintiff to maintain an action alleging the following facts: After ordering Mr. Ricks to the hospital for a seriously infected hand, Dr. Budge refused treatment and walked out because Mr. Ricks would not immediately catch up on his past due accounts. This decision is frequently cited by commentators for the proposition that it is illegal to abandon a patient who cannot pay. However, these facts do not support a general prohibition of economic abandonment. Instead, the holding is perfectly consistent with purely "procedural" abandonment law, which only requires the doctor "to give the patient sufficient notice so the patient can procure other medical attention if he desires," id., and prohibits patient abandonment only at a critical stage in the course of treatment.

Additional support for this view is suggested in the most recent leading abandonment decision, Payton v. Weaver, 182 Cal.Rptr. 225 (1982). There, the court allowed a physician to stop treating an uncooperative patient despite the unavailability of any substitute care. This case concerned a renal dialysis patient who "frequently appear[ed] for treatment late or at unscheduled times in a drugged or alcoholic condition, used profane and vulgar language, and on occasion engaged in disruptive behavior, such as ... cursing staff members with obscenities." Although Dr. Weaver's attempts to find alternative treatment centers were unsuccessful, the court held that he "gave sufficient notice of [his intent to cease treatment] and discharged all his obligations." It is impossible to determine, though, whether *Payton v. Weaver* invokes a purely procedural abandonment rule because its compelling facts might also provide substantive justification for the decision to discontinue treatment.

Finally, in Muse v. Charter Hosp. Winston–Salem, Inc., 452 S.E.2d 589 (N.C.App.1995), aff'd mem., 464 S.E.2d 44 (N.C.1995), the court ruled that a psychiatric hospital illegally interfered with the physician's medical judgment when it encouraged the discharge of an adolescent patient whose insurance ran out, which led to the patient's suicide three weeks later. Although the opinion never mentions the abandonment doctrine, it is based on the hospital's alleged "policy or practice" of discharging patients when their insurance runs out. Even so, the decision is subject to the same uncertainty as *Ricks* and *Payton*: we don't know whether the hospital is liable because the discharge policy is *per se* wrong or because of the procedure it followed in failing to sufficiently notify the parents of their son's fragile condition so they would be sure to find alternative care. Even with such notice, however, a patient who is discharged for financial reasons is likely to have a difficult time finding alternative care.

B. THE LEGAL CONTENT OF THE TREATMENT RELATIONSHIP

The balance of this chapter addresses the legal doctrines that arise once a treatment relationship is formed: confidentiality, informed consent (including conflicts of interest), and contractual modification of treatment obligations. The physician's duties under each of these doctrines are shaped by the fiduciary nature of that relationship.

1. The Fiduciary Core of the Treatment Relationship

"Fiduciary" relationships exist in a number of legal and social realms. Fiduciary duties arise as heightened aspects of general tort and contract law rather than through a separate branch of legal doctrine. Fiduciaries must meet high standards of loyalty, diligence, and solicitude in carrying out their legal obligations. Black's Law Dictionary 625–26, 298 (6th ed. 1990) is instructive: "scrupulous good faith and candor"; the responsibility to act "primarily for another's benefit" in connection with a duty undertaken; the subordination of one's personal interests to that of another; a relationship founded on the "trust or confidence" one person reposes in "the integrity and fidelity" of another who, as a result, can exercise "domination and influence"; the "highest standard of duty imposed by law"; trusteeship. A slightly weaker form of fiduciary status exists in what is called a "confidential relation," which arises when "on the one side there is an overmastering influence, or, on the other, weakness, dependence, or trust, justifiably reposed." Contrast these notions with normal arm's-length market relations.

In the treatment relationship, a patient, often dependent and diminished by illness, seeks care from a professional with a complex body of knowledge and skill essential to the patient's well-being and perhaps to life itself. He entrusts his care to the doctor, which often requires the sharing of intimate knowledge and deep invasions of physical and emotional privacy. These and other characteristics clearly bring it within the ambit of a fiduciary relation, and courts have consistently so held. "The patient's reliance upon the physician is a trust of the kind which traditionally has exacted obligations beyond those associated with arms-length transactions. His dependence upon the physician for information affecting his well-being, in terms of contemplated treatment, is well-nigh abject." Canterbury v. Spence, 464 F.2d 772 (D.C.Cir.1972). These characteristics form common underpinnings for the legal doctrines explored in the balance of this chapter.

2. Confidentiality

Confidentiality is a core element of the fiduciary content of the treatment relationship. This section explores the values it protects, the means by which the law safeguards it, and the tensions it creates in competition with other values.

a. The Duty to the Patient

So basic is the expectation of confidentiality in medical treatment that patients and health-care providers alike generally assume it will be honored, without ever specifically discussing it (though clinical psychologists routinely announce at the outset of therapy that certain information may require its breach). Confidentiality is a foundational principle of medical ethics, recognized in both the Hippocratic Oath ("Whatsoever I shall see or hear in the course of my profession ... if it be what should not be published abroad, I will never divulge, holding such things to be holy secrets") and the AMA Principles of Medical Ethics ("A physician shall ... safeguard patient confidences within the constraints of the law.")

The main rationale for honoring medical confidentiality is utilitarian. Confidentiality is thought to encourage individuals to seek medical care who might otherwise avoid doing so out of shame, embarrassment or fear of disclosure of their affliction; this benefits the sick, the currently well (in providing reassurance about similar protection for the treatment of their own future illness), and society as whole in the form of improved public health. The philosopher Sissela Bok identifies three additional, more generally applicable, reasons for honoring confidentiality: a recognition of the interest in autonomy over personal information; the legitimacy of not only *having* secrets, but of *sharing* them (i.e., respect for disclosure and relational intimacy); and the special obligation that arises from the act (where it occurs) of having *promised* not to disclose. Sissela Bok, Secrets 119–24 (1982). For these reasons, the duty of confidentiality is protected through a variety of legal sources.

(1) Common Law Protections.

Redress for providers' unauthorized disclosure of patient information has been sought using theories including infliction of emotional distress, malpractice, breach of a confidential relationship or of fiduciary duty, invasion of privacy, and breach of contract. *See* Humphers v. First Interstate Bank of Oregon, 696 P.2d 527 (1985) and cases discussed therein. This variety probably reflects uncertainty, in particular jurisdictions, as to what theory is best adapted and likeliest to prevail, but strategic considerations may also be at play, relating to whether expert testimony is needed (as in a malpractice claim), the availability of damages and the existence of damage caps, and comparative limitations periods. Where the claim is brought in tort, courts may require that an enforceable *duty* of confidentiality be established by reference to sources of settled law or policy, and will look to the professional ethical standards noted above, as well as to the jurisdiction's various statutory provisions, for evidence of that duty and its limits.

(2) Statutory Protections.

Many state licensure laws provide that a breach of patient confidence constitutes unprofessional conduct that will subject a physician to discipline or license revocation. Such laws vary as to whether the violation must be intentional or whether a merely negligent disclosure will suffice, and they generally acknowledge that other provisions of law may create exceptions.

In addition, most states have evidentiary rules which prohibit certain health care providers (generally doctors or psychotherapists) from disclosing patient confidences. These "privilege" rules generally apply only to testimony, and to the discovery and/or admissibility of records, in judicial proceedings. Accordingly, they confer only limited protection of patient confidentiality. Even in litigation there is variation in the classes of professionals to whom they apply (see, e.g., Buchanan v. Mayfield, 925 S.W.2d 135 (Tex.App. 1996) (privilege inapplicable to communications with dentist)), they are easily waived by the patient, and they are subject to many exceptions. There is no physician-patient privilege in the Federal Rules of Evidence, although the Supreme Court recently implied a psychotherapist-patient privilege under Rule 501, Jaffee v. Redmond, 116 S.Ct. 1923 (1996).

Disease (or subject)-specific statutes creating confidentiality duties have expanded in recent years. Many states have HIV-protective statutes, enacted out of concern over discrimination and ostracism of HIV patients. Federal law imposes confidentiality requirements on records of patients in federally-assisted drug and alcohol treatment programs, 42 USC § 290dd–2. More than half the states have recently enacted legislation addressing the discriminatory use of genetic information by insurers or employers, and there is some federal regulatory law on the subject; there is a great deal of debate concerning the adequacy of protection of genetic information more generally. As with any protective law, the precise reach of these statutes is sometimes uncertain. E.g., Doe v. Marselle, 675 A.2d 835 (Conn.1996) ("willful" disclosure of HIV information means knowing or intentional, as opposed to inadvertent, but does not require intent to cause harm to the patient).

The patchwork nature of these various protective laws, and the increasing proliferation and computerization of medical information, have prompted ongoing efforts to craft a comprehensive medical privacy law, possibly at the federal level.

b. *The Duty to Protect Third Parties and the Limits of Confidentiality*

In some circumstances a health care provider owes a duty to parties *outside* the treatment relationship, arising from an important interest or value in competition with the duty to the patient. Failure to meet this competing duty may result in civil or even criminal liability, and fulfilling it sometimes (but not inevitably) requires a breach of patient confidentiality. Broadly speaking, the applicable rules may be broken into three categories, two statutory and one common law.

(1) Statutory Duties to Report

The most common and time-honored exception is the required reporting of various communicable diseases to state public health authorities. The list of conditions varies somewhat from state to state but AIDS, and in many states HIV infection alone, have been added in recent years. In a similar category fall reports of child and elder abuse, alcohol and drug abuse, and, in some states, uncontrolled epilepsy among licensed drivers. Where the reportable condition is not uniquely dependent on medical diagnostic expertise, the statutory duty may run to other health care providers, and sometimes laypersons, as well; in those instances the tension with a duty of confidentiality may be reduced or eliminated. The purpose of all such requirements is to enable authorities to protect identified individuals or the community at large.

These reporting statutes sometimes explicitly grant the provider immunity from liability to the patient for any resulting breach of confidence. Such immunity is readily implied in any event, where the patient's condition unambiguously meets a clear reporting obligation. (Of course, notwithstanding this immunity, as a practical matter the treatment relationship may well be fractured by the mandated disclosure). Under some statutes, *failure* to report can result in civil or criminal sanctions, and doctors who do not report might be found *per se* liable to anyone who is injured.

A second class of mandatory reporting exists for knife or gunshot wounds that appear to be non-accidental. Here the policy is generally to catch and punish wrongdoers, rather than to protect third parties against continuing or future harms. One might argue that this constitutes a less compelling basis for the breach of confidentiality. On the other hand, the instrumental *purpose* of protecting confi-dentiality—encouraging treatment—may be dam-aged to a lesser degree in the case of such violent injuries, since the victims (like those in any emer-gency) may be highly likely to obtain treatment out of necessity.

(2) Common Law Duty to Protect Third Parties

Even absent a statutory duty, a legal duty to protect third parties might arise through the com-mon law whenever the patient's condition poses a significant risk or danger to others. Tarasoff v. Regents of University of California, 551 P.2d 334, 340 (Cal.1976). Examples include patients with con-tagious diseases, violent psychiatric patients, and persons with medically-related driving impairments. It is often extremely difficult to resolve these situa-tions under the common law. The existence and scope of the duty to third parties is often unclear; moreover, in those cases where this duty competes with the obligation of confidentiality, the tension is likely to be very great and immediate, and the consequence to the treatment relationship of a breach of confidence quite destructive. It is often the case that a physician has no legally safe course available.

Note at the outset that, although these common law cases are frequently described as imposing a duty to *warn* third parties, the category is better conceptualized as a duty to *protect* third parties, since there may be steps other than direct warning that are necessary or sufficient to discharge the duty. Such steps may not require breaching confidentiality.

Broadly speaking, physicians are liable for harm to a third party if three conditions are met: (1) there is a known or reasonably foreseeable hazard, arising in some way from the physician's patient; which (2) places at risk one or more foreseeable (though not necessarily individually identifiable) third parties, of whom the plaintiff is one; and (3) the provider failed to take a reasonable course of protective action. The first condition may be thought of as giving rise to the *existence* of the duty; the second determines the party(ies) to whom the duty is *owed*; and the third defines the *scope* of the duty.

(a) Basis of the Duty: "Hazard" or "Special Relationship"

The familiar basic tort rule is that one has no duty to take protective action on another's behalf simply because one recognizes (or should recognize) that the other is in avoidable jeopardy. Courts have historically recognized exceptions for "special relationships" that give rise to a duty to control someone's conduct for the benefit of a third party (e.g., hospitals' relationships with mental inpatients). *See generally* Restatement (Second) of Torts §§ 314, 315 (1964). In practice (though often without careful explanation), courts have found a protective duty in somewhat broader and varied circumstances, employing mixed rationales of patients' dangerousness and physicians' ability to take protective steps; hence the choice of the word "hazard" in the above typology, rather than "special relationship."

The cases include physician relationships with non-hospitalized patients with contagious diseases (in which courts have imposed a duty to warn caregivers and family members of their risk) (*see* Bradshaw v. Daniel, 854 S.W.2d 865, 871 (Tenn. 1993) (reviewing cases)); dangerous psychiatric outpatients (beginning with the famous case of *Tarasoff, supra,* which, though novel because it applied the duty to protect third parties to a psychotherapist with a dangerous outpatient, actually relied on the contagious disease outpatient cases just mentioned as precedents); and patients with medical conditions that impair their driving ability. Some modern courts suggest that *any* physician-patient relationship is "special" and triggers a protective duty, without reference to the type or degree of hazard. *Tarasoff, supra*; *Bradshaw, supra*. This formulation imposes an open-ended physician duty to protect third parties against hazards of any kind. Also, where the physician actually *creates* the hazard, as for example in providing medication that temporarily impairs driving ability, courts sometimes eschew the need to find a "special relationship."

Very recently, a few courts have moved beyond the requirement that the patient present some personal physical hazard to a third party, holding instead that the physician's duty is triggered merely by learning or suspecting that someone else is in danger, from whatever source. Thus in *Bradshaw v. Daniel*, 854 S.W.2d 865 (Tenn.1993), where a man died from a *non*-contagious disease (Rocky Mountain Spotted Fever), the court nonetheless held his physician had a duty to warn the man's wife, who subsequently also died from the disease, that she too was at risk based on the fact that the ticks that transmit the disease to humans tend to "cluster." Two recent cases, harbingers of a rapidly emerging issue, have found that physicians have a similar protective duty running to family members of individuals with heritable genetic conditions. Safer v. Estate of Pack, 677 A.2d 1188 (N.J. Super. 1996) (physician may have duty to warn family members);

Pate v. Threlkel, 661 So.2d 278 (Fla.1995) (duty to family members recognized; dischargeable by advising patient). This problem is especially complex given the potential tension between such a protective duty and a "right *not* to know" that many persons may assert in order to avoid the emotional implications of confronting their susceptibility to a family history of genetic problems. To resolve the tension perhaps physicians will need to develop generic questions for family members about their wish to acquire genetic knowledge based on family history, in advance of any actual disclosures— though even doing that much may well breach the patient's confidence or a right not to know.

The health care provider's duty to accurately detect, or diagnose, the hazardous condition is measured by a professional negligence standard— whether the provider "knew or should have known" of the condition and its dangerousness—an inquiry that normally requires expert testimony. In the *Tarasoff* context (psychiatric violence), many psychiatrists and psychotherapists doubt the profession's, and their own, ability to predict dangerousness accurately. The standard, however, does not require an *accurate* prediction, but only one arrived at *non-negligently*—i.e., through adherence to professional standards of care.

The continuing extension of a duty to protect third parties may be animated by the "rescue" ethos discussed in sec.A.2.b, *supra*: in some situations a third party's protection simply exerts a sufficiently strong moral claim that courts will recognize a duty to act, notwithstanding traditional tort rules and the strong competing value of patient confidentiality.

(b) Foreseeable Plaintiffs

The physician's duty, once recognized, runs to reasonably foreseeable plaintiffs. In many cases this will be only one, or a few, persons of known identity. For example, with psychiatric dangerousness there is frequently a threat to a specific individual (*Tarasoff*). With contagious disease, family members or caregivers may be the primary persons at risk. In such cases, the imminence of the harm and the reasonableness of imposing the protective duty are perhaps the clearest and the most readily understood.

However, the individuals in the class of prospective plaintiffs need *not* be actually known, or even personally identifiable, in all cases. An impaired driver, for example, threatens all other drivers, passengers and pedestrians on the road. It is *not* the case, however, that a physician's duty to protect third parties runs to the world at large; there will generally be some limit of reasonableness under the circumstances that identifies the extent of the protected class. Indeed, this variation in *who* must reasonably be protected is related to the final element: *how* protection is to be accomplished.

(c) Discharge of the Duty to Protect

Recall that steps short of breaching patient confidentiality may often suffice to meet the physician's protective duty. For example, an elderly patient with badly impaired vision may be privately persuaded by the physician to relinquish his car keys; an HIV-positive patient may be instructed regarding safe sex or abstinence and the avoidance of needle sharing; a man with a genetic condition might be told of its familial nature and left to his own judgment with respect to family disclosure. On the other hand there are certainly cases where the protective duty might *only* be met by a breach of confidentiality: a vision-compromised patient who will not voluntarily stop driving; an HIV-positive patient who refuses to adopt safe sexual practices; or a psychiatric patient who intends to harm a former lover. Here the duty of confidentiality and the duty to protect come unavoidably into conflict, generating a Scylla and Charybdis of competing legal obligations.

Even here, the precise *form* in which confidentiality is broken may well vary with the circumstances, and "warnings" to specific individuals may be neither necessary nor useful. In the case of the vision-impaired driver, the physician might talk to the spouse or children or call the motor vehicle division, but it would be impossible (and thus vain) to "warn" all other drivers and pedestrians. In the case of the HIV patient, the physician might contact the HIV patient's lover or call the state health department (which, in some states, then assumes responsibility for "partner notification" or other contact tracing). Indeed it is especially logical for state public health authorities to take over the duty to protect in the context of transmissible diseases like HIV, since there may be multiple partners or exposed individuals, whose identity the physician could not reasonably be charged with knowing or ascertaining. In the case of the psychiatric patient, the physician might directly warn the potential victim or contact the police. As *Tarasoff* recognized, discharge of the protective duty—even where it necessarily involves the breach of confidentiality— does not require a warning *per se,* but instead requires "whatever . . . steps are reasonably necessary under the circumstances."

This, of course, is not entirely reassuring, given the ambiguity of what constitutes the "correct" choice and the potential liability for either decision. This is an area where it would be helpful for the law to confer qualified immunity to providers who, in good faith, follow *either* course. Thus a physician would be protected against both the patient's claim of breach of confidentiality and the third party's claim of failure to protect by a "buffer" rule that required him only to demonstrate (for example) careful consideration, investigation of options, and perhaps an (anonymous) ethics consultation, with respect to the most advisable course of conduct. Some state legislatures have enacted just such a rule in the specific context of HIV-related behaviors. The rule might be extended legislatively to other subjects. Alternatively, in common law litigation, a court might judicially create such an immunity—or, if it believed one outcome superior to the other, could nonetheless announce a liability rule *prospectively* so as to avoid unfairness in the initial case.

3. Informed Consent

Probably no medico-legal doctrine has received more scholarly attention in the past several decades than the law of informed consent. This is due in part to its central role in defining the legal content of the treatment relationship.

The core value underlying the law of informed consent is autonomy. By requiring a physician to disclose information meant to enable the patient to choose knowledgeably among reasonable medical alternatives, informed consent seeks to place patients in control of the course of their medical treatment. The rules reflect the agency principles that underlie fiduciary law: the physician is agent who supplies information and advice to patients, enabling them to decide what treatment to order according to their personal preferences and interests.

It is commonly observed that there is considerable tension between the doctrine and aspirations of informed consent law as articulated and advocated by judges, lawyers and legal scholars committed to autonomy, and the real world of medical practice which recognizes competing values (such as beneficence) and, in many cases, doubts the efficacy of informed consent law to achieve its goals. Core assumptions can be questioned as an empirical matter, including patients' capacity to absorb the relevant information, whether people actually desire to make their own medical decisions, and the degree to which autonomy is cherished as the primary value in medical decisionmaking (among different groups and cultures, as well as by particular individuals). Informed consent claims appear to play a fairly small role in overall litigation against physicians for medically-induced harms, and are rarely brought independently of an accompanying malpractice claim alleging that the care actually delivered was substandard. Nonetheless the doctrine is important, both for its formal contribution to the law "on the books" and because it is one of the tools through which the content of the treatment relationship is negotiated.

a. Classic Doctrine

Informed consent derives from the intentional tort of battery, but modern informed consent law in almost all jurisdictions is fundamentally a negligence-based doctrine. To recover, a patient must typically show that: (1) the course of treatment followed carried with it an undisclosed risk; (2) the physician's nondisclosure of that risk breached the applicable standard of care owed to the patient; and (3) the undisclosed risk caused the patient's injury, in both a physical sense (by materializing) and a behavioral sense (in that, with proper disclosure, the patient would have made a different treatment choice, thus avoiding the harm). The following discussion briefly surveys these elements. The other essential preconditions for a valid informed consent are that the patient must have the requisite mental capacity, and consent must be voluntary. Note at the outset that the presence or absence of medical negligence in the *performance* of treatment is irrelevant to the claim; informed consent rests on a separate theory, and separate proof.

(1) Risk: What Information Must Be Shared?

Generally speaking, physicians must disclose the patient's diagnosis; the nature, purpose, and probability of success of the proposed treatment; the salient risks accompanying the treatment, including risks arising from the patient's particular medical susceptibilities; and the alternatives, including *their* risks, consequences, and probability of success. One hopes that these are precisely the issues that all physicians consider when deciding the best course of treatment, so requiring physicians to convey this to their patients follows directly from the doctrine's theoretical goal of giving patients the benefit of their physicians' superior knowledge and expertise. In reality, however, physicians, like others who practice in a complex profession, do not deliberate explicitly on each factor that might influence each decision. Instead, they adopt "clinical heuristics" or rules of thumb which embed many implicit assumptions, so that informed consent doctrine might alter how physicians think as well as what they say. In reality, it does not often do either, since these disclosures are usually made in writing on forms written or approved by lawyers and long since forgotten by the physician.

(2) Negligence: Measuring the Physician's Conduct

Two main rules have developed for assessing the adequacy of the physician's disclosure. A slight majority of states apply a "professional" standard: the physician must disclose information that would be shared by a reasonably competent physician in comparable circumstances. This approach, of course, is quite analogous to the legal requirement for medical or surgical *performance* in malpractice cases, and has the same central characteristic: the law, in searching for a standard, defers to (normative) medical practice. In informed consent litigation this approach is disadvantageous to patients in two senses. First, as with malpractice, it generally requires expert testimony to prove both what the applicable professional standard of disclosure is, and to establish that it was breached. Second, there is no relief if the professional standard does not happen to call for disclosure; patient informational expectations, however reasonable, are theoretically irrelevant.

Some commentators have argued, and some courts have held, that the medical profession itself in recent years has adopted sufficiently patient-oriented disclosure norms that disclosures will routinely be adequate even under the professional standard. Others defend the "professional" rule on the view that it protects a physician's judgment about how to properly allocate time between informational disclosure and medical or surgical treatment (though that tension is not an inevitable one, since nonphysician providers can also disclose and counsel). In any case there is this irony in the professional standard: a remedial doctrine, founded on the perceived need to enhance autonomy, defers to the collective judgment of those whose behavior generated the need for reform.

A smaller number of jurisdictions adopt a "patient-oriented" disclosure standard, which measures the adequacy of physician disclosure not by normative physician practices but by patient needs: all information "material" to the decision of a "reasonable patient" must be "unmasked." Canterbury v. Spence, 464 F.2d 772 (D.C.Cir.1972). The core of this approach is the notion that, once armed with the requisite information, the decision about what medical course to follow is a personal, value-laden, nontechnical one, rather than one dependent upon medical expertise. Many commentators believe this rule better reflects the autonomy-based essence of the doctrine.

This lay-oriented standard avoids the need for expert testimony on the adequacy of disclosure. However, expert testimony may still be needed on causation and on whether the undisclosed information constitutes a risk of, or an alternative to, the treatment. States following this approach generally apply an objective ("reasonable patient") standard of materiality, rather than a subjective ("this patient") one; this is designed to avoid holding physicians liable for failing to accurately guess the unknowable informational needs of particular patients. (Courts say this is consistent with the "foresight" rather than "hindsight" requirements of "orthodox negligence doctrine." *Canterbury.* Query, though, whether it makes sense to measure—as this rule does—the adequacy of A's conduct by the *expectations* therefor of a "reasonable B.") Moreover, it is not obvious how providers are to decide, in advance, that a particular risk would be "material" to even a "reasonable" patient; by its nature, this standard leaves many questions for the jury, which entails great uncertainty for providers.

(3) Causation

There are two dimensions of causation in an informed consent case. First, the patient must actually be harmed by the undisclosed risk. Proof of this often requires expert testimony. Second, the plaintiff must show that the risk's disclosure would have led to a different medical decision, thereby avoiding the harm. This non-technical question does not require expert testimony. Most courts ask whether a "reasonable" (rather than *this*) patient would have made a different medical choice, in order to avoid the hazards of self-serving, *post hoc* patient testimony; in this approach the patient's own testimony may be relevant but not dispositive. One can argue, though, that the usual vehicles for truth-ascertainment (cross-examination, the existence of prior inconsistent statements, testimony of knowledgeable others and the like) would adequately counter this risk, and that the choice of this objective-patient standard takes away much of the autonomy that the doctrine otherwise promises.

(4) Exceptions to the Duty to Disclose

In several circumstances courts have recognized (often in dictum) exceptions which, in essence, privilege nondisclosure. It is generally the physician's burden to prove such a privilege or defense. By and large these exceptions are narrowly construed because of their capacity to undercut the doctrine. They include, first, undisclosed risks that are "common knowledge," and second, risks of which the particular patient is already aware. There is also no duty to disclose in emergencies, particularly where the patient is incapacitated, though even here "proxy" consent by relatives is advisable. Some courts also recognize a "therapeutic" privilege, when disclosure of the usual information would be so damaging or upsetting emotionally that it would "menace" the patient's well-being. *Canterbury*, however, cautions against broad recognition of such a principle lest it swallow the rule, and against the medical paternalism of invoking it as a means of imposing "needed" treatment on the patient that the physician fears would be rejected if fully described. Finally, a few courts have observed in passing that autonomy, taken seriously, allows waiving the right to informed consent, since only an ironically paternalistic view of informed consent would *force* the doctrine's customary vision of autonomy on an unwilling patient.

b. Conflicts of Interest and Fiduciary Principles

Though courts very often *characterize* the treatment relationship as a fiduciary one, their actual reliance on fiduciary doctrines to impose liability has been somewhat selective. However, in a famous case the California Supreme Court held that a physician must disclose economic or research interests "unrelated to the patient's health" that might affect the physician's judgment. Moore v. Regents of the University of California, 793 P.2d 479 (Cal. 1990). The court noted that this result is supported both by informed consent law, and more directly by the conflict of interest prohibition imposed by fiduciary law. In *Moore*, the physician had an interest in developing biotechnology products from cells taken from the patient's diseased spleen. The court held this should have been disclosed prior to surgery and during post-surgical care, especially since some of that care had no direct therapeutic purpose.

Fiduciary doctrine also influenced a ruling under ERISA (which incorporates trust law) that a managed care company must disclose to its members the financial incentives it uses to influence primary care physicians' decisions about when to refer to specialists. Shea v. Esensten, 107 F.3d 625 (8th Cir.1997). Fiduciary or informed consent doctrine might also require these financial disclosures from physicians, although this has never been done under traditional fee-for-service arrangements, which create incentives to over-treat. However, those incentives are more obvious. Fiduciary law sometimes considers a conflict of interest to be so debilitating that it is prohibited regardless of disclosure and consent. Chapter 1.D.3.b discusses which financial arrangements in medicine are currently banned by regulatory law.

c. *Emerging Applications of Informed Consent*

Traditional informed consent cases involve medical or surgical risks. In recent years, courts have also been asked to include in the disclosure obligation novel kinds of risks, such as the risks of doing nothing, the economic factors just mentioned, or particular traits of the individual physician. These cases generally arise in "patient-oriented" jurisdictions since the materiality standard allows much more freedom to innovate than does professional custom.

Truman v. Thomas, 611 P.2d 902 (Cal.1980) is the leading ruling that informed consent applies to a patient's refusal of a diagnostic test. The court sent to the jury a case where the physician failed to impress upon his patient forcefully enough the potential consequences of foregoing the Pap smear he offered to her. In this "informed refusal" situation, the risk arises from the *lack* of a medical procedure rather than its performance. Physicians complain that this rule sets no limits on how aggressive they must be in convincing reluctant patients.

Another developing area is the disclosure of a physician's individual skills. In one recent case a surgeon performed a complex and risky surgery to clip a patient's brain aneurysm, which went poorly resulting in quadriplegia. The patient did not pursue either surgical negligence nor nondisclosure of the risks of the procedure, but instead argued that the physician wrongfully withheld information (and may have actually provided misleading answers to the patient's questions) about his lack of personal experience performing this procedure. Evidence indicated, but the patient claimed not to know, that less experienced physicians have higher surgical morbidity and mortality and that a more sophisticated and resource-intensive hospital was available within 90 miles as an alternative site. The court ruled these considerations are material to a reasonable patient's decision and upheld the trial court's admission of this evidence under that theory. Johnson v. Kokemoor, 545 N.W.2d 495 (Wis.1996). Physicians complain that this ruling tends to keep less-senior practitioners from gaining necessary experience and might stigmatize even senior practitioners who attract the most difficult cases, which are more prone to complications. This will become increasingly controversial as more provider-specific outcomes measures become available.

A related and sensitive topic is disclosure of personal, non-technical physician characteristics. An

HIV-infected physician offers a riveting test case. The statistical risk of a doctor transmitting HIV is extremely low, but public anxiety over the possibility is understandably high, and the consequences of infection are devastating. One decision struck the balance in favor of the patient, requiring an HIV-positive surgeon to disclose his status. Behringer v. Medical Center at Princeton, 592 A.2d 1251 (N.J. Super.1991). Similar questions arise for physicians with substance abuse problems. Physicians argue that these issues are better resolved through hospital privileging decisions, medical licensure, professional ethics, or the threat of malpractice litigation.

In a significant decision pointing the opposite direction, the California Supreme Court affirmed a jury finding that physicians are not bound to disclose a cancer patient's (short) life-expectancy in order to enable him to put his financial and business affairs in order. The court held that, despite the physician's fiduciary status, informed consent law does not require disclosure of risks to nonmedical interests nor of everything a patient might literally want to know. Arato v. Avedon, 858 P.2d 598 (Cal.1993). Considering that California is historically among the most liberal jurisdictions in developing and applying the doctrine, this case is an indication of the law's ambivalence about the future scope and application of informed consent law.

4. Modifying the Terms of the Treatment Relationship

Recall that the formation of the treatment relationship is essentially contractual in nature. Once established, however, tort and fiduciary law generally govern the parties' conduct and their mutual obligations. This section explores the extent to which patients and physicians are free to modify those rules and define the terms of their relationship in accordance with their own preferences.

Courts have generally refused to enforce agreements with patients by which health care providers try to waive their liability for negligence. The leading case is Tunkl v. Regents of the University of California, 383 P.2d 441 (Cal.1963), in which the California Supreme Court concluded that a hospital's exculpatory agreement with a patient, signed at admission, bore all the indicia of an unconscionable adhesion contract.

Tunkl and similar cases do not, by their terms, preclude liability waivers that fall short of full exculpation, and in fact courts are likely to enforce releases from liability where the care provided departs from standard medical practice for good reason, as when a patient leaves the hospital early against medical advice, or refuses recommended medical treatment. In this connection, consider Shorter v. Drury, 695 P.2d 116 (Wash.1985), holding that a document signed by a Jehovah's Witness surgical patient, releasing providers from responsibility for consequences "due to my refusal to permit the use of blood," constituted an enforceable assumption of the risk of an otherwise-avoidable death, rather than an unenforceable exculpation of negligence.

Courts have also responded favorably to agreements changing the forum or mechanism of dispute resolution. For example, HMOs may require their members to arbitrate rather than litigate medical negligence claims, at least where this is agreed to through bargaining by a powerful representative (a large employer) and there is a choice of alternative plans. Madden v. Kaiser Foundation Hospitals, 552 P.2d 1178 (Cal.1976). *But see* Cannon v. Lane, 867 P.2d 1235 (Okla.1993) (contrary result). On the other hand, "point of treatment" arbitration agreements, presented for signature upon hospital admission or at the doctor's office, are less likely to receive judicial approval because of concerns about their fairness, though these decisions too are not uniform.

Agreements to *alter* the prevailing standard of care, rather than to waive it entirely as in *Tunkl*, are more difficult. If notice is adequate and there is some choice, should HMOs (for example) be allowed to contractually bind enrollees to accept a lower-than-normal standard of care (e.g., anything above "gross negligence") by plan providers, as a cost-containment mechanism that would benefit enrollees by reducing premiums? The law on such questions is not well-developed, but is likely to be a focal point of controversy as medical standards are increasingly subsumed within managed care contractual arrangements. For competing arguments, see Clark Havighurst, Health Care Choices: Private Contracts as Instruments of Health Reform (1996) (endorsing such a contractarian approach); Maxwell

Mehlman, *Fiduciary Contracting: Limitations on Bargaining Between Patients and Health Care Providers,* 51 U. Pitt. L. Rev. 365 (1990) (criticizing it).

PART II

THE LEGAL STRUCTURE OF HEALTH CARE DELIVERY

The health care industry, historically a staid and stable enterprise, is currently in tremendous ferment as a consequence of the cost containment pressures described in Chapter 1. These pressures have caused unprecedented experimentation with new organizational forms and relationships that do not fit easily into preexisting legal categories. As a consequence, whereas a generation ago hospitals and doctors could, aside from malpractice suits, get along quite nicely with little more legal advice than occasional tax consultation, health care corporate and regulatory law is now a flourishing practice area that requires sophistication in subjects as diverse as antitrust, facility licensure, insurance regulation, and labor law. The materials in the second part of this book examine these and other private and public law doctrine that have the greatest relevance to the unique legal problems presented by the structure and functioning of the contemporary health care delivery system.

CHAPTER 3

HOSPITAL STRUCTURE AND REGULATION

The prototypical health care institution is the general, acute care, medical-surgical hospital. Hospitals come in many shapes and sizes. Most are private and non-profit, although many are run by government entities or owned by investors. Some are quite small, with 50 beds or less; others are 1000-bed behemoths. Community hospitals offer more basic services such as routine child birth and simple operations while major medical centers and teaching hospitals strive to have the most comprehensive and state-of-the-art programs and technology available. Other hospitals specialize in only a limited range of medicine, such as mental health or cancer. Nevertheless, hospitals of all types share important common features. There are also common features among all medical institutions. Although we seldom mention nursing homes, home health agencies, diagnostic clinics, and ambulatory surgery facilities in this book, often times when we refer to hospitals we could equally well include these other medical facilities. Finally, the border between health care insurance and health care delivery is rapidly fading due to innovative arrangements like HMOs, which are both service facilities and financing vehicles. Therefore, many of the laws that affect traditional facilities also apply to HMOs or to joint ventures between doctors and hospitals.

This chapter explores the basic legal environment in which traditional hospitals and other health care facilities are organized and operated. It addresses the bodies of law that are most familiar to health care lawyers, and for the most part it regards these facilities in their simplest structure. Although this chapter considers the obvious extensions of this basic legal doctrine to HMOs and other more complex ventures, most of the cutting-edge legal developments that respond to these innovative structures are taken up in the subsequent chapters.

A. HOSPITAL AND FACILITY REGULATION

1. Licensure, Certification, and Private Accreditation

Hospitals and other health care facilities such as nursing homes are so heavily regulated that they are sometimes thought to approach the status of a public utility. One hospital once toted up that it must submit reports to and comply with rules set by over three dozen government authorities and a half dozen private bodies. The primary authorities are: 1) state licensure, 2) private accreditation, and 3) certification for participation in government insurance. These three sources are each legally distinct, but their substance and processes are intertwined to a considerable extent.

Since the mid century, virtually every state has regulated the operation of hospitals, nursing homes, and similar facilities through licensure statutes and regulations. Hospital licensure provisions typically read like a gigantic building code for the hospital industry, specifying a host of architectural, safety, and sanitation minutia as a condition for issuing or renewing an operating permit.

Private accreditation of hospitals and other health care facilities overlaps to a significant extent the function performed by state licensure. The Joint Commission on Accreditation of Healthcare Organizations (formerly, "of Hospitals"), which is referred to as (the "JCAHO" or the "Joint Commission") is a private accreditation body maintained jointly by the AHA, the AMA, and two other physician groups. Its accreditation standards impose detailed organizational and procedural standards for the structure and operation of each hospital department. The JCAHO wields enormous authority and influence because virtually no hospital of respectable size risks the business consequences of jeopardizing its accreditation status. Many states effectively delegate their licensing function to the JCAHO by incorporating its standards by reference.

Similarly, hospitals and other facilities must be certified as fit to participate in Medicare and Medicaid, under standards very similar to those for licensure and accreditation. Accordingly, the federal Medicare program automatically deems all JCAHO-accredited hospitals as meeting certification standards for participation. One can question whether it is an appropriate public policy to abdicate regulatory oversight to the industry itself, but "deeming" has been upheld as constitutional. Cospito v. Heckler, 742 F.2d 72 (3d Cir.1984). Certification standards are somewhat more demanding for nursing homes under Medicaid because this has been seen as an area were traditional state oversight mechanisms were lax. In response to litigation, see Estate of Smith v. Heckler, 747 F.2d 583 (10th Cir. 1984), HHS has imposed an extensive set of regulations that govern in considerable detail the treatment plans, living environment, legal rights, and human dignity of nursing home patients. They are enforced primarily through state licensure officials.

This overlapping regulatory structure raises a host of legal issues, only a few of which will be touched on here. (Among the omitted issues are constitutional and procedural challenges to adverse decisions.) The first issue is jurisdiction. Facility licensure typically excludes physician offices under the premise these fall under the jurisdiction of physician licensure. But, when is a physician's office really a facility? Consider, for instance, freestanding emergency centers ("FECs"), colloquially known as "Doc-in-Boxes." These store-front medical clinics cater to no-wait, no-appointment medical needs of an urgent nature, short of life-or-limb threatening conditions. They provide a convenient and less expensive alternative to hospital emergency rooms for conditions such as broken legs, bad cuts, and sudden illnesses. It can be argued that FECs are nothing more than glorified doctors' offices, which traditionally have not been covered by facility licensing laws. However, states are beginning to amend their statutes to cover these and other novel delivery arrangements such as ambulatory surgery clinics.

A second set of issues concerns how these regulatory authorities attempt to define and oversee the quality of care. Public policy theorists distinguish among three different ways to measure quality of care: *structural measures* such as corporate and managerial organization and the composition of relevant committees; *process measures* such as protocols and forms that must be followed by professional staff to avoid mistakes and catch errors; and *outcomes measures*, which look at how patients are actually doing. Critics charge that licensing, accreditation, and certification are directed almost exclusively to structural and process measures, which produces an excessive focus on red tape and busy work for administrators.

Attempts to invoke bottom-line outcomes measures are underway, such as infection rates, death rates, and patient satisfaction, but they encounter persistent difficulties over the methods of measurement and comparison, so that low-scoring facilities are not unfairly penalized by bad luck or because they happen to attract more difficult or serious cases. Both the Joint Commission and the Medicare/Medicaid certification standards now require that hospitals and other institutions adopt outcomes measures of quality, as does the National Committee on Quality Assurance (NCQA), which accredits HMOs. Ultimately, however, this push for outcomes measures may devolve into another set of structural or process measures. Licensing and accrediting organizations find it difficult to impose any absolute performance standards, since numerous factors, many out of the facility's control, affect how patients actually do. Therefore, most of these new standards require simply that facilities take and monitor these performance measures, not that they achieve any particular score.

2. Certificate of Need Laws

A more specialized regulatory regime that exists in most states requires hospitals and other health care institutions to obtain a certificate of need ("CON") from a government agency before constructing new facilities, purchasing major medical equipment, or instituting new health services. CON laws arose from the National Health Care Planning and Development Act of 1974, 42 U.S.C. § 300k (repealed), which required states to adopt CON regulation in order to receive certain federal health care funding. In 1987, though, Congress became disenchanted with the CON regulatory approach (for reasons explained below) and repealed the federal mandate, leaving states free to depart from the federal model. Consequently, a number of states have scrapped their CON laws entirely and a number of others have substantially loosened their regulatory reigns. Still, CON has a significant presence in the majority of states and is expected to remain as a permanent fixture in the health care regulatory apparatus for some time to come.

Certificate of need laws are a response to the excess capacity in capital resources. Hospitals commonly have far more space than they require, frequently operating at 50 percent capacity or lower. The hospital industry is also notorious for its redundancy of technology: if one hospital acquires the latest technological gadget—formerly, a CAT scanner, later a magnetic resonance imager (MRI), and now a positron emission tomographer (PET)—then immediately all of the other hospitals in town set about making duplicative purchases. The same is true for glamorous services such as heart transplant programs.

Ordinarily, market forces penalize such overinvestment of capital resources because a firm with excess capacity must charge higher prices to service its debt or to provide a competitive return on investment equity. More conservative firms are then capable of quickly undercutting the high spender, resulting in a net decrease in income. In health care, however, higher prices do not automatically cause a loss of business under traditional, open-ended, cost-or charge-based reimbursement.

A second inflationary factor in capital spending is the nonprofit status of much of the hospital industry. The only use that charitable hospitals are permitted to make of their earnings is to plow them back into the facility. The prestige of non-profit managers is measured not by the profitability of the enterprise but by its size and presence in the community. This leads to what is sometimes called the hospital industry's "edifice complex"—an almost obsessive desire to build and spend.

If all we faced were a single layer of fat atop an otherwise lean hospital industry, our problems would not be so severe, but an important phenomenon amplifies the effect of this profligate capital spending. Health care appears to be ruled by what is known as "Roemer's law," which states that empty beds generate increased demand for services. Roemer was the first to identify and explain the apparent paradox that health care utilization tends to be the highest where there is the most unused capacity. When hospitals expand, they urge their medical staffs to think of more inventive ways to use the facilities, and once the facilities are fully used, hospitals expand once again. The fundamental point of Roemer's law is that more than the costs of bricks and mortar are at stake: capital expenditures drive up operating costs, which lead to increased reimbursement and then further expansion, in a never-ending spiral.

CON laws are designed to curb these excesses by requiring hospitals and other health care facilities (such as nursing homes, ambulatory surgery clinics, and home health agencies) to demonstrate a need for new projects that involve a substantial expenditure. The exact expenditure thresholds and project descriptions vary widely from state to state, but generally speaking the amounts involved must be $1 million or higher.

Hospitals have found various inventive means for circumventing the reach of CON regulation. The most prominent technique is to arrange a new project under the auspices of a physician rather than a hospital because most CON laws apply only to health care institutions and specifically exclude expenditures by physicians in private practice. In one case, a group of doctors was successful in purchasing without approval a magnetic resonance imager, a multimillion dollar piece of sophisticated diagnostic equipment usually found only in major medical centers. Boulware v. State, Dept. of Human Resources, 737 P.2d 502 (Nev.1987). However, some states have amended their statutes or regulations to encompass projects of this nature that are intended to serve hospital patients.

When a project—say, the construction of a new hospital—is subject to review, the controversy shifts to how the need for additional hospital capacity (measured by number of beds) is properly determined. Bed-need methodology is usually spelled out, either in a State Health Plan or in CON regulations, in a manner that establishes a mathematical formula for comparing the existing stock of beds with the projected demand. For instance, a simple formula might call for a maximum of 4 beds per 1000 population in a designated geographical region. A more refined formula might set the ratio according to the historical utilization experience of each local population group to account for differences in age or health, or might use more sophisticated techniques to account for the net migration of patients in and out of the geographical area.

If these mathematical formulae fail to establish a net shortage of hospital beds, CON applicants frequently attack the formulae as being unreasonably rigid and tending to ignore other, less quantitative statutory factors such as the quality of services proposed and the increased accessibility to underserved groups. While such attacks are difficult to maintain, *see* Statewide Health Coordinating Council v. General Hospitals of Humana, 660 S.W.2d 906 (Ark.1983), they have enjoyed surprising success in some jurisdictions.

A CON applicant's task is far from over when it identifies an underserved pocket of population. Typically, such an applicant will find itself fending off several other competing applications. These comparative hearings can quickly degenerate into disputes over trivia such as who has the superior parking lot design or who is cutting down the fewest trees. Procedural complexities also abound in the CON review process, so that the process is often lengthy and expensive.

For these and other reasons, several studies have demonstrated that CON regulation has virtually no effect on health care investment or expenditures. This failure is due primarily to several shortcomings in the design and implementation of CON laws. Even as designed, CON laws are very limited in scope. First, they address only the major capital *costs* of health care; hospitals are still free to *charge* whatever they want, and they are free to release their spending pressures in other directions such as salaries and other operating costs. Second, "need" for new facilities is usually measured in terms of current—*i.e.*, inflated—treatment patterns. Therefore, CON laws at best remove only the outer layer of fat, that is, the existing excess capacity; they are inherently incapable of reversing the built-in inflationary base of treatment intensity caused by the "Roemer cycles" of past decades. Moreover, CON laws are constitutionally incapable of eliminating increases in service intensity. With "need" as the primary focus, it is impossible to turn down any new facility or technology that provides a conceivable benefit.

CON is more than simply a failed attempt, though; it may have produced net harms. Most obvious are the costs of administering a complex and broad-based regulatory program. Less obvious, but more troubling, are the anticompetitive effects of limiting market entry by new hospitals. Prohibiting new construction absent a showing of need protects established hospitals from competition by new firms that desire to enter overbuilt markets, the very markets where competition is the most needed. Moreover, where new construction is warranted, it has sometimes been observed that CON regulators play favorite to local hospitals over newcomers in choosing among competing applicants. This is not entirely the result of dirty pool; the more established applicant is inherently able to expand at the lowest cost. It is for this reason that certificates of need serve almost like franchises in perpetuity: once a hospital has a foothold in the market, it is in the naturally favored position to continue to expand to meet future growth in need. This protectionist character of CON laws explains why the hospital industry strongly supports this form of regulatory control.

B. HOSPITAL AND HMO MEDICAL STAFF ISSUES

1. Medical Staff Structure and Staff Selection Process

The hospital medical staff is an institution unique to North America. Elsewhere in the world, hospitals employ a select group of specialist physicians who practice exclusively in a single hospital under a salaried arrangement. In the United States (and Canada), the tradition has developed that virtually all physicians practice in more than one hospital and they do so independently of the hospital. Doctors are neither paid by hospitals nor do they pay for the privilege of using hospital facilities. The relationship between doctor and hospital is symbiotic, each sustaining the other through an implicit exchange of benefits—the hospital provides a doctor's workshop and the doctor provides a supply of patients.

This fundamental division between hospital and doctor pervades the health care delivery system. A hospital patient (or her insurance company) will receive a bill for physician services that is separate from the bill for hospital services. Medicare is split into two parts, Part A for hospital (and other institutional) costs and Part B for physician charges. Blue Cross/Blue Shield plans, which are the largest component of the health insurance industry, reflect the same dichotomy.

The only formal manner in which hospitals and doctors interact is through the hospital medical staff. The medical staff is the collection of doctors that enjoys admitting privileges at a hospital. The significance of "admitting privileges" is understood only by realizing that, in a formal sense, hospitals do not admit patients directly; instead, they receive patients that are admitted by practitioners on the medical staff. Thus, although American hospital medical staffs are much more "open" than their European counterparts, it is not the case that literally every doctor may admit patients to every hospital. Only those practitioners who meet the criteria established in the hospital's medical staff bylaws are allowed to join.

The medical staff bylaws are an organizational document that is separate from the hospital bylaws. JCAHO accreditation standards emphasize that the staff bylaws may not be amended unilaterally by the hospital (or by the medical staff). The medical staff's effective veto power over selection criteria further reinforces physicians' control over the credentialing process that is explained in the following section. These organizational patterns developed by custom in the early twentieth century and became formally institutionalized in the mid-century through the standards set by the JCAHO.

In addition to admitting privileges, medical staff membership also determines "clinical privileges," that is, which department of the hospital a physician is allowed to join and what procedures within that practice area the physician may perform. Also, there are various categories of staff privileges that reflect the degree of regularity of a physician's practice at the hospital: active staff, courtesy staff, and visiting staff.

The process of selecting and periodically reevaluating medical staff members is referred to as "credentialing" or "peer review." Because hospital credentials are based on the practitioner's medical competence, the hospital delegates much of the evaluation and decision making authority to the existing medical staff members themselves (hence the name "peer review"). For new applicants, various medical staff committees first conduct a fact-gathering process and the staff then votes and sends its decision to the hospital board of governors as a recommendation, which the board usually accepts. Existing staff members are reviewed every two years through a more streamlined process. If either review process produces an adverse finding, the initial or renewal applicant is entitled to a formal, evidentiary hearing to contest the finding. If the finding is sustained, the hospital can revoke, suspend, or limit the privileges of existing staff members.

There are three important qualifications to the generalized medical staff model that has just been depicted. First, physicians are not the only medical professionals that potentially can hold staff privileges at a hospital. Beginning in 1984, the JCAHO accreditation standards were revised to allow hospitals to admit psychologists, nurse midwives, chiropractors, podiatrists, and other so-called allied health professionals—licensed medical practitioners whose practice areas are restricted to some limited segment of medicine. The second qualification relates to certain hospital-based specialists. Hospitals usually find it convenient to employ or contract exclusively with a limited number of radiologists, anesthesiologists, pathologists, and sometimes emergency room physicians. Unlike most practicing doctors, these hospital-based physicians typically do not admit patients and they have direct financial arrangements with the hospital, either as partners, independent contractors, or employees. Finally, teaching and government hospitals depart from the traditional American model by employing large portions of their medical staffs.

Another important development is the replication of the medical staff structure within other medical institutions, particularly, within HMOs. Although HMOs do not give physicians the same autonomy over financial matters or the content of the bylaws, they do replicate the credentialing and peer review processes in deciding which physicians to admit to and retain in the network. Accordingly, many of the issues raised in this chapter with respect to hospitals also exist for HMOs, but in a somewhat altered legal framework.

2. Economic Credentialing, Exclusive Contracts, and Institutional Control

Some hospitals have grown increasingly disenchanted with the traditional medical staff model under which physicians remain financially and organizationally autonomous from the institution. These hospitals have attempted to fundamentally restructure themselves into a more classically hierarchical structure in which practicing physicians are subservient to top administrators. (Naturally, there are both physician and lay administrators.) For the most part, they have been largely unsuccessful because of the numerous ways in which the independent medical staff is firmly institutionalized both in practice and in law. Legally , medical staff independence is virtually assured because it is written into the existing corporate bylaws. Most courts have ruled that medical staff bylaws constitute a contract that cannot be unilaterally amended by the hospital administration. Even if this were not the case, altering the traditional arrangement might be found to violate JCAHO accreditation standards, which are embodied in licensure and certification law.

Failing wholesale restructuring, hospitals have attempted to accomplish de facto restructuring by inserting new criteria into the bylaws that define medical staff membership, or by circumventing the medical staff credentialing process through exclusive contracts. These efforts are discussed under the term "economic credentialing." The gist of this term is to call attention to the effort to use economic criteria as well as quality of care criteria to determine physicians' relationship with the hospital. For instance, a hospital might attempt to exclude from the staff or terminate the contract of a physician who consistently loses money on their Medicare or HMO patients.

When hospitals take the direct route of attempting to amend the formal bylaws, they usually do not succeed. If they cannot convince the existing staff to vote in favor of these changes, courts have held that the hospital lacks authority to unilaterally amend the bylaws or to make medical staff decisions outside of the authorized credentialing process. However, hospitals have adopted a different technique with more success, using exclusive contracts. They have limited clinical privileges in specified departments to select physicians or groups under contract with the hospital, as is traditionally done with hospital-based physicians. When a physician's contract is terminated or given to someone else, the physician often complains that there has been a de facto termination of medical staff membership. A number of courts have responded, however, that contract termination leaves medical staff privileges unaffected. Since contracting naturally falls within the purview of hospital administration, hospitals are able through this technique to limit hospital access using any criteria they wish.

How is this legal position sustainable? Courts draw the technical distinction between the honorific or status aspects of possessing medical staff membership versus the practical opportunity to exercise these privileges. Only the former, they reason, is subject to the credentialing process; the latter is under the control of hospital administration. This may appear at first to be an unconvincing hypertechnical distinction, but courts reason it has something of substance. Physicians with staff privileges can still enjoy the reputational benefits of this status, even if they have limited access to the hospital. And, hospitals must be afforded some opportunity to control physical access lest some clinical areas becomes overcrowded or uncoordinated. Consider, for instance, a hospital that allowed any physician who wanted to work in a hospital emergency room at any time. Sometimes, there would be no one there; other times, the emergency room might become like a crowded bazaar in which physicians vie for each new patient who enters the door. On the other hand, this characterization is clearly exaggerated.

In any event, economic and administrative issues are expected to influence medical staff decisions much more explicitly in the future. *See generally,* M. Hall, *Institutional Control of Physician Behavior: Legal Barriers to Health Care Cost Containment,* 137 U.Penn.L.Rev. 431, 518 (1988). When they do, courts will confront whether the substance of the decision is legitimate. So far there has been very little actual litigation on the merits. One of the few decisions remotely on point, Knapp v. Palos Comm'y Hosp., 465 N.E.2d 554 (Ill.App.1984), held that it is permissible to exclude a physician for ordering too many tests and doing too much surgery, but that case focused on the medical risks of unnecessary care, not on the economic costs. No case to date that considers the merits cleanly sustains a hospital's exclusion decision based on criteria unrelated to, much less opposed to, the quality of patient care. However, this is becoming commonplace for HMOs.

3.   HMO Deselection and Managed Care Contracting.

One has to wonder how health care institutional terminology initially takes hold and later evolves. One such puzzle is the term "deselection." This has become the accepted term to refer to decisions by HMOs to drop physicians from their networks. Naturally, this is beginning to produce considerable litigation, as physicians claim they are dropped for no good reason, or for reasons contrary to the public interest such as advocating too strenuously for their patients or objecting to HMO policies they think are wrong.

At the outset, HMOs avoided the dilemma they saw hospitals in when confronting economic credentialing. Rather than allow medical staff decisions to be made only by a physician-controlled credentialing process, HMOs parallel processes which they can choose between. HMOs sometimes use a classic credentialing process focused on quality of care, but they also write into the physician contracts the explicit right of either party to invoke "no-cause" termination. This allows an HMO to drop a physician without any explanation when it prefers not to air its true reasons. This also allows physicians to leave the HMO without penalty if they are dissatisfied.

Physicians who are dropped unceremoniously in this fashion allege in lawsuits that no-cause terminations are used to cover up nefarious HMO motives. For instance, HMOs have been accused of dropping physicians whose race or location brings in less desirable patients. In response, courts have split in their rulings. Some courts simply enforce the contractual arrangements as written. Others impose a public policy override, which refuses to let HMOs drop physicians for reasons contrary to the public interest or that would breach the implied covenant of good faith and fair dealing. The leading decision is Harper v. Healthsource New Hampshire, 674 A.2d 962 (N.H.1996), which sustained a cause of action against an HMO that dropped a physician without explanation, where the physician alleged the real grounds related to differences of opinion over patient care policies. The law here is influenced by the judicial limitations in recent years to the common law "at will" employment doctrine. This public policy limitation allows physicians who make the proper allegations to obtain a hearing on the actual reasons for termination. They bear the burden of proof, however, and they must show reasons that are more than just arbitrary or mistaken. This is a more demanding showing than that required under the body of law discussed in the next section that governs hospital medical staff disputes.

Before turning to that topic, it is worth considering why "no-cause" termination clauses are so common in HMO physician contracts. One might think that physicians would strenuously object to including these because they shift so much power to the HMO, and so their presence signals that the HMO has disproportionate bargaining power. This is undoubtedly true in some instances, but in others physicians insist on including these clauses. They often enter HMO contracts somewhat wary about how things will turn out and therefore eager to be able to withdraw quickly and easily. Also, if the HMO were to want to terminate them for quality of care reasons, they would much prefer a less explicit process and one that does not result in having to report the action to the National Practitioner Data Bank.

As for the issue of bargaining power, in many markets HMOs feel that physicians have the upper, or at least an equivalent, hand. Most physicians contract with HMOs on a nonexclusive basis and so physicians can shift their allegiances similar to the influence they wield over competing hospitals (although they lack the same ability to take their patients with them when they switch HMOs). Accordingly, they are often in a position to negotiate aggressively with HMOs that recruit them to their networks. This is especially true for popular physicians whose patients will select insurance plans based on their membership in the network.

When negotiating managed care contracts, several other important issues arise in addition to no-cause termination. Primarily, physicians must read these contracts with care to determine what payment and treatment terms they are agreeing to. Often, managed care contracts are written in a manner that gives the HMO carte blanche to bind the physicians to any payment and coverage terms they happen to negotiate with employers or other purchasers. Another controversial issue is liability. These contracts often use indemnification clauses to shift all liability for medical outcomes to the physician, even though some bad outcomes may result from the HMO's own decisions about which treatments are covered.

4. Hospital Medical Staff Disputes

a. Introduction

Long before the HMO deselection controversy, hospitals found themselves in the confluence of several strong legal and economic currents affecting the medical staff relationship. Under the tort law development known as "hospital corporate liability," a hospital (and potentially its medical staff) is responsible to its patients for the quality of the physicians allowed to practice within the institution. Darling v. Charleston Comm'y Mem. Hosp., 211 N.E.2d 253 (Ill.1965). However, a strong opposing force exists by virtue of the increasing economic

importance to physicians of medical staff membership. Access to a hospital is essential to carry on
almost any form of medical practice. Physicians who
are excluded from the major hospitals (and often
there is only one hospital in a community) have
their entire professional practice at stake. Moreover, physicians view it as essential to have access
to several hospitals in order to compete more effectively for a supply of patients, particularly in recent
years with the physician market experiencing what
some consider a "glut" of doctors.

Nevertheless, if these were the only interests at
stake in medical staff selection, it would be puzzling
if courts were to concern themselves greatly with
physician complaints about the merits of negative
membership decisions. Excluding a qualified physician runs counter to a hospital's fundamental economic interest because hospitals obtain patients
mainly through their medical staff members. This
economic motive would be expected to serve as an
effective check against hospitals screening doctors
with excessive zeal. The flaw in this supposition is
that staffing decisions are not entirely based on the
institution's interests. The existing medical staff,
which has tremendous influence over these decisions, has a precisely contrary interest: it stands to
lose business when new members are admitted to
the staff. This built-in economic bias creates a risk
that meritorious physicians will be excluded for
reasons unrelated to patient care.

Given the intersection of these three sets of powerful interests—the institution's, the physician ap-

plicant's, and the existing medical staff's—it is not surprising that medical staff disputes have boiled over into the courts in great numbers, second only in the medical/legal arena to malpractice litigation. The remainder of this section examines the judicial response to these challenges under the common law. ("Exclusion" refers to either the denial of an initial application or the revocation of existing staff privileges.) Antitrust theories are reserved for Chapter 4.

b. Theories of Judicial Review

A variety of conventional causes of action are available to an excluded physician, but each of these theories is limited in some significant respect. A doctor might allege a violation of due process and equal protection rights under the Constitution, but this theory is limited to *public* hospitals—those owned or operated by state or municipal authorities. *See* Blum v. Yaretsky, 457 U.S. 991 (1982). At a private hospital, a doctor might contend that his dismissal from the staff violates contractual rights of process and substance contained in the medical staff bylaws. However, this theory is not available to new applicants who have not yet been admitted to the staff, and some courts have rejected this theory altogether. Under tort law, excluded physicians can allege defamation or tortious interference with contract, but these theories are also laden with various elements that restrict their application to staff exclusion decisions generally.

Federal statutory law protects against discrimination in the workplace. Courts divide on whether medical staff membership is the functional equivalent of employment. Regardless, this law reaches only discrimination based on race, sex, religion, national origin, or disability. State law is beginning to offer medical practitioners somewhat greater relief through statutory provisions in several states that impose requirements of procedural and substantive fairness on hospitals. Most notably, some states prohibit discrimination based on a practitioner's medical degree, school of practice, or nature of license. These statutory protections remain spotty, however. Consequently, excluded practitioners have sought innovative common law theories that provide more broad-based scrutiny of the procedural and substantive fairness of private hospital peer review.

Excluded physicians have principally attempted to rely on a novel theory that characterizes private hospitals as public facilities. The pathbreaking case is Greisman v. Newcomb Hospital, 40 N.J. 389, 192 A.2d 817 (1963). There, the hospital maintained a policy requiring all staff members to hold an M.D. degree, which excluded Dr. Greisman, an osteopath, from consideration. The court acknowledged that Newcomb Hospital was a private facility and therefore not subject to constitutional constraints; nevertheless, it imposed a *common law* duty of fairness in the medical staff selection decision based on its finding that hospitals constitute a "quasi-public" facility. This is a sharp departure from the principle of free association that is deeply imbedded in our market-based economy, according to which private enterprises ordinarily can decide to do business or not with anyone they like for any reason, absent invidious discrimination or antitrust violation.

The *Greisman* decision attracted much academic attention and a notable following among other state courts. However, several states have refused to adopt the quasi-public characterization of their private hospitals. Conceptually, the problem is in identifying what characteristics should appropriately render a private business "quasi-public" and thus subject to such regulation. The New Jersey court relied on a body of now obscure law. These cases originated from ancient precedents in 15th century English common law that treated common carriers and innkeepers as "businesses affected with the public interest," thereby imposing on them unique public service duties of fairness in their terms of service and prohibiting discrimination against classes of customers. This area of the common law fell dormant around the turn of the century as it became subsumed by statutory regulation of public utilities. Nevertheless, *Griesman* found that these common carrier precedents still apply in the modern context.

These old cases generally applied to common callings that enjoyed monopoly status. For instance, in 15th century England, inns typically were spaced evenly along the roadway at the distance of one day's journey and only one ferry operated at a local river crossing. Sometimes, these common callings also enjoyed support from the sovereign through an exclusive royal charter. These characteristics were viewed as justifying special duties of public service because, if these businesses arbitrarily denied services, the customer would have no alternative source.

Likewise, Newcomb Hospital in the *Greisman* case had effective monopoly status since it was the only facility in the area. And the hospital received ample government support through construction grants, tax exemption, and county funding of indigent care. It might be objected that common carrier law protected only the rights of customers (*i.e.*, patients), not employees (doctors), but the court was careful to observe that, because patients obtain hospital admission only through staff physicians, the discrimination against Dr. Greisman was in effect discrimination against his patients.

However, there are important objections to the quasi-public theory, some of which the courts have articulated and some of which they have not. First, the key characteristic for public facility status in other areas of the law seems to be the *natural* monopoly character of the enterprise. Railroads, telephone companies, and the public utilities have all been regulated as public facilities because of the belief that they were natural monopolies. While single-hospital communities are certainly common, this is far from the necessary or even predominant industry pattern. Where there are several competing hospitals, or where there is the *possibility* for hospital competition, it is unclear why hospitals require any greater policing than private business decisions in any other important industry.

Second, if public service duties are imposed, this does not extend protection to all physicians, only those attending physicians with primary authority over patient admissions. This limitation would keep the doctrine from applying to hospital-based physicians such as radiologists and pathologists. Third, once the common carrier precedent is invoked, it would seem necessary to follow all of the ramifications of that precedent, which leads to some surprising and unsettling results. Why stop at physician staff membership; what about other employees? Why stop at admission policies; what about general patient care policies? Observe that ancient English courts scrutinized not only the customer selection policies of common carriers but also the prices they charged. Even more startling, realize that common carriers were held strictly liable for the injuries they caused. These possibilities have not yet been explored in the courts, but they remain pregnant with potential for imaginative plaintiffs' counsel.

c. *The Scope of Judicial Review*

In states where judicial review is available under the public facility theory, the controversy then shifts to the scope or intensity of review. In *Greisman,* for instance, the court held that a policy excluding all osteopaths is illegal because osteopaths are licensed by the state to practice the full range of medicine and the hospital presented no evidence that osteopaths as a group provide inferior care. The court ruled that it is illegal "to preclude an application for staff membership, not because of any lack of individual merit, but for a reason unrelated to sound hospital standards and not in furtherance of the common good." This statement leaves a number of unanswered questions, though: Are any general, class-based distinctions among practitioners valid, or must anyone with a relevant license be considered on their individual merits? If some general criteria are allowable, what degree of evidence or justification is required to establish the validity of such criteria? And what procedural safeguards are required to insure that criteria are reasonably applied in particular cases?

Greisman encourages hospitals to review physicians on their individual merits. In doing so, what criteria validly count toward merit? The courts, in answer to this question, have articulated a number of legitimate and illegitimate considerations. It is proper to require personal references, to insist on adherence to medical staff rules, to require residence near the hospital, and to require a minimum level of malpractice insurance. It is not proper to require membership in the local medical society or to require references from current members of the medical staff. The harm of the latter criteria is that they give incumbent physicians the power to "black ball" new arrivals to the community.

When a medical staff takes adverse action against an individual physician based on legitimate considerations, say, lack of professional competence, the court then must determine how closely to scrutinize the evidence supporting that decision. Courts have expressed extreme reluctance to second guess the informed judgment of medical professionals. Representative is this frequently quoted statement:

> No court should substitute its evaluation of such matters for that of the Hospital Board.... Human lives are at stake, and the governing board must be given discretion in its selection so that it can have confidence in the competence and moral commitment to its staff. The evaluation of professional proficiency of doctors is best left to the specialized expertise of their peers, subject only to limited judicial surveillance.... In short, so long as staff selections are administered with fairness, geared by a rationale compatible with hospital responsibility, and unencumbered with irrelevant considerations, a court should not interfere.

Sosa v. Board of Managers, 437 F.2d 173 (5th Cir.1971).

This deferential attitude does not apply uniformly in all medical staff disputes, however. When there is reason to be suspicious that an asserted ground for exclusion is in fact a disguise for personal animosity or bias, the courts have exercised much more stringent review. A good example is the standard of review for staff discipline based on alleged personality problems. Courts have sustained the exclusion of a doctor with a history of rancor and disruption since poor relations among the staff may impair the quality of service provided the patient. However, medical staff disharmony often grows out of a doctor's legitimate criticism of hospital policy or of other doctors' performance, or it might have its basis in personal or economic matters wholly unrelated to medical policy. Therefore, other courts have balked at the exclusion of physicians simply on the basis of their inability to work with others on the staff; they have required some greater, more specific showing that this inability directly jeopardizes patient care.

Greisman might be read to preclude any rejection of a medical staff applicant other than on an assessment of the practitioner's individual competence. This reading is clearly too broad, however. "Courts should sustain a hospital's standard for granting staff privileges if that standard is rationally related to the delivery of health care." Nanavati v. Burdette Tomlin Memorial Hospital, 526 A.2d 697 (N.J. 1987). The problem in *Greisman* is that the hospital made no attempt to justify a rational basis for excluding osteopaths. Suppose the hospital had observed that M.D.s, as a lot, are marginally better than D.O.s because most osteopaths failed to get into regular medical school. Would that be sufficient to justify the discrimination? Or would it be sufficient to contend that osteopaths subscribe to a different school of practice and the hospital wished to limit itself to practitioners who all hold the same treatment philosophy?

The answer depends on what degree of scrutiny a court chooses to inject into a review of "rationality." Although constitutional principles do not apply to private hospitals, it still may be helpful in understanding the common law fairness doctrine to recall the analytical framework that courts have developed in their equal protection jurisprudence. Class-based discrimination against a school of practitioners might be reviewed under a "minimum scrutiny" standard of rationality, which would accept almost any plausible explanation for an exclusionary policy, or it might be scrutinized under a more heightened "intermediate" level of review that requires substantial justification if there is some reason to be suspicious of the medical staff's motives. (A "strict scrutiny" standard that required a "compelling interest" would be inappropriate unless the hospital employed a "suspect classification" such as race, gender or national origin.)

Most courts have refused to accept justifications for the exclusion of osteopaths of the sort just suggested, thus evidencing an intermediate level of review. However, other courts have sustained discrimination against osteopaths with very little justification. *E.g.,* Hayman v. City of Galveston, 273 U.S. 414 (1927) (finding no equal protection violation in a state hospital's exclusion of osteopaths); Stern v. Tarrant County Hosp. Dist., 778 F.2d 1052 (5th Cir.1985) (en banc) (upholding exclusion of osteopaths, over a vigorous dissent that condemned "the bigotry of an allopathic-dominated state hospital district that refuses to be bothered by either the state law, the federal constitution or the facts").

Courts have also reached conflicting results over whether a hospital can discriminate on the basis of medical certification. In contrast with excluding incompetent doctors, a hospital may want to limit staff membership to only the most highly qualified doctors, as designated by "board certification," which some courts find permissible. The indirect effect of this requirement, however, may be to exclude certain schools of practitioners who do not meet the eligibility requirements, practitioners such as osteopaths. Therefore, other courts have struck down these policies as discriminatory.

The great bulk of case law addressing medical staff disputes concerns the required elements of procedural fairness for denying or revoking staff privileges, rather than the substance of those decisions. Much of this body of law has essentially the same content as general administrative law (even though private hospitals are not subject to the Administrative Procedure Act or the Constitution), so it will receive only cursory discussion here. This law is now largely determined by the federal statute discussed below which creates a qualified immunity for peer review participants if the process is conducted fairly. The statute and its regulations detail the procedural components necessary to qualify for this immunity, which essentially codifies the existing state caselaw. Procedural steps are also usually specified to some extent in the medical staff bylaws.

Generally speaking, hospitals must provide physicians a formal evidentiary hearing before taking any final adverse action on either expulsion or admission. In the case of initial applicants, this hearing normally occurs as a review of the hospital board's initial decision to deny the application. In the case of revoked or suspended privileges, the hearing usually occurs once an initial decision is made to consider taking disciplinary action against the physician. Prior to the hearing, the hospital must give the doctor adequate notice of the charges and evidence against him. The doctor must be allowed to appear and present contrary evidence. Members of the hearing panel must not have had prior exposure to the case or otherwise have formed a biased or predetermined position on the merits. (The latter prohibition may be particularly troublesome in small rural hospitals, where it may be necessary to use a hearing panel composed of persons from outside the hospital.) In other respects, these hearings need not be conducted with the formality of a courtroom proceeding. For instance, most courts agree that lawyers can be excluded from the proceeding and that the hearing can be conducted without cross examination.

5. Physician Membership in Managed Care Networks

As noted above, these same issues exist with respect to physician membership in managed care networks such as HMOs, but the legal framework differs to some extent. At the outset, one might ask why HMOs should have to engage in further credentialing, considering that physicians are already screened by licensing authorities and several hospitals. As a practical matter, this debate is moot since HMOs have decided to do this voluntarily, perhaps prompted by the threat of corporate liability, and credentialing is generally required by HMO licensing laws and by HMO accreditation standards. The issue then arises what legal protections physicians have when they are excluded.

The legal focus so far been entirely on the removal of existing network members, which is known as "deselection," rather than on the denial of initial applicants. In part, this is because the available legal theories don't support initial applicants to the same degree as with hospitals, and in part because HMOs are not viewed or established in the same open staff model as are community hospitals. But, this area of law is still in development.

First, consider whether the quasi public facility characterization should apply to HMOs. The case is much weaker than for hospitals, since HMOs are much less likely to be monopolistic, and there is a lesser degree of government support. Intuitively, the public does not regard them in the same light as a community institution that should be open to every physician, nor do they usually hold themselves out in this manner. Therefore, most courts decline to extend the hospital precedents to HMOs. So far, only California differs, and there the issue is presently under review by its Supreme Court. Potvin v. Metropolitan Life Ins. Co., 63 Cal. Rptr. 2d 202 (Cal. App. 1997), review granted, 67 Cal.Rptr.2d 1 (July 30, 1997).

Other courts, however, have adopted a different legal theory for judicial scrutiny of HMO staffing decisions. They have applied the employment at will precedents discussed above to contract terminations that violate public policy. Where this cause of action exists, how does the resulting level of scrutiny differ from under the quasi-public facility theory? First, note that the at-will contract theory applies only to existing network members, not to applicants. Second, note that the theory explicitly allows "no-cause" terminations. The burden is on the excluded physician to show there was a hidden bad cause that is contrary to public policy. Reasons that are merely arbitrary or poorly supported, which would violate quasi-public review, are permissible under this theory. What does in fact violate public policy? Retaliating against physicians who stand up for patients' rights, similar to the "whistleblower" cases discussed below, is a prime example. But, it would appear that economic grounds or personality disputes, even if manifestly unfair, are permissible because they don't contravene established public policy.

Finally, as for process rights, HMO physicians, like hospital staff members, have a right to receive the process that is promised in their contracts, but, as noted above, managed care contracts frequently contain no-cause termination provisions that allow immediate dismissal for no stated reason.

6. Peer Review Confidentiality and Immunity

Courts adjudicating medical staff disputes have been reluctant to interfere in the internal workings of a hospital or HMO, both because they feel unqualified to make judgments about medical competence and because they fear that such litigation will deter physicians from performing their vital peer review role effectively. Intensive peer review is considered essential to improving the quality of medical care, a matter of heightened concern as a result of the medical malpractice "crisis." Therefore, a number of state and federal enactments clothe the medical peer review process with confidentiality or immunity.

a. State Peer Review Confidentiality Statutes

Some states have "shield laws" that provide a degree of legal immunity for hospital peer-review committee members and witnesses by protecting them, for instance, from defamation suits. A greater number of states have a peer review *confidentiality* statute that protects the proceedings of any hospital peer review committee from discovery, and a few decisions have found a common-law basis for such a privilege even in the absence of such statutes. This peer review privilege shields internal hospital review records both in actions *by* the sanctioned doctor (for improper exclusion) and in actions *against* the doctor (for malpractice). However, these statutes prohibit disclosure only of information and reports that are generated by internal review committees; they do not entirely remove relevant information from the litigation process if the information is derived from independent, noncommittee sources.

b. Federal Peer Review Immunity

The federal Health Care Quality Improvement Act of 1986, 42 U.S.C. § 11101 *et seq.*, confers sweeping peer review immunity, but of a highly qualified sort. On first reading, this Act would seem to render irrelevant much of the discussion in this and the next chapter, for it states that "any person who participates with ... [medical peer review] action shall not be liable in damages under any law of the United States or of any State" except for civil rights laws. *Id.* § 11111. However, there are many important exclusions from and limitations to this immunity.

First, this federal peer review immunity applies only to decisions involving physicians; it does not shield decisions to exclude other medical professionals. Second, even for physicians, the law is concerned only with the exclusion of individual physicians; immunity does not attach to the establishment of general credentialing criteria that exclude groups of physicians. Third, even for individual physician exclusions, the Act covers only exclusions based on conduct that could adversely affect the health of a patient, omitting decisions based on economics or on more general ethical concerns or the welfare of the institution.

Even for those cases that do meet the Act's definition of "professional review action," immunity attaches only if the exclusion decision "meets all the standards specified [in the Act]." *Id.* These detailed procedural and substantive standards in essence track much of the law that the Act attempts to preempt. To qualify for immunity, a peer review action must be taken:

> (1) in the reasonable belief that the action was in the furtherance of quality health care, (2) after a reasonable effort to obtain the facts of the matter, (3) after adequate notice and hearing procedures are afforded to the physician involved or after such other procedures as are fair to the physician under the circumstances, and (4) in the reasonable belief that the action was warranted by the facts.

Id. § 11112.

Because of these limitations, many of the medical staff cases mentioned in this chapter and in chapter 4.B (antitrust boycott law) would fail to qualify for immunity under the Act. Even for those that would, the impact of the Act is less than one might first think. A physician challenging an exclusion will still allege that the hospital's or HMO's action was not in good faith, was not supported by substantial evidence, and did not comport with fair procedures, all of which allegations, if true, would disqualify the defendants from the immunity. Thus, the substantive core of these disputes has simply been shifted to the outset of the case. However, this shift has the important procedural effect of lessening the defendants' burden of proof: "A professional review action shall be presumed to have met the [required] standards ... unless the presumption is rebutted by a preponderance of the evidence." *Id.* The statute also contains a fee shifting provision that penalizes frivolous challenges to peer review decisions. *Id.* § 11113. Finally, it is important to note that the statute immunizes only damages actions, not actions for injunctive relief.

C. LABOR AND EMPLOYMENT LAW

Labor and employment law is an area of emerging significance to health care institutions, not only because these topics are important to all industries, but also because these topics contain dimensions that are unique to the health care setting. Unlike most industries where the interests at stake are simply the employee's right to a job and the employer's right to do business as it sees fit, here the courts must consider how the law should be shaped to accommodate the additional concerns of avoiding disruption in medical services. Moreover, precedents drawn from conventional employment contexts are sometimes not easily transferrable to the independent character of licensed medical professionals.

1. Labor Law

a. Patient Care Concerns

The law of collective bargaining provides the clearest examples of the unique problems that medical employment raises. The National Labor Relations Act ("NLRA"), 29 U.S.C. § 151 et seq., establishes a comprehensive regulatory scheme, administered by the National Labor Relations Board

("NLRB"), to protect employees' rights (1) to form a union, (2) to require their employer to bargain with the union in good faith and honor collective bargaining agreements, and (3) to strike if they are dissatisfied with the terms or conditions of their employment. Prior to 1974, nonprofit hospitals were not subject to this Act, but in that year Congress added provisions directed specifically to the health care industry. 29 U.S.C. §§ 152, 158, 169, 183. In doing so, Congress expressed a concern that union activity not disrupt hospitals' important patient care mission. Specifically, both the Senate and the House expressed concern that too many unions within a single institution would pose an excessive risk of crippling, repetitive strikes: "Due consideration should be given by the Board to preventing proliferation of bargaining units in the health care industry." 1974 U.S.Code Cong. & Ad.News 3950.

Incorporating this "nonproliferation" mandate into labor law has proven troublesome. The controversy turns on how the NLRB should frame its test for determining the proper definition of a hospital bargaining unit. Normally, the NLRB makes unit determinations according to a "community of interests" test, that is, whether there is such a close community of interests between, say, RNs and LPNs to include them both in the same union. However, in response to a series of reversals holding that this test did not give sufficient weight to the nonproliferation mandate, the NLRB adopted a "disparity of interests" test for the health care field. This test creates a presumption in favor of the largest possible unit that does not include employees with clearly disparate interests. Some circuits, however, criticized or refused to enforce the disparity of interests test. In order to resolve all the confusion, the NLRB, which is notorious for deciding all policy issues in adjudication, took the extraordinary step of initiating a rulemaking proceeding to define the proper approach to health care unit determinations. Its final regulations allow up to eight separate bargaining units: RNs, physicians, other professionals, technicians, clerical, maintenance, security guards, and others. 29 C.F.R. § 103.30, 54 Fed.Reg. 16336 (April 21, 1989). These rules generated intense opposition from health care management, which perceives that carving units into smaller divisions greatly increases the ease of unionizing and therefore is inconsistent with the nonproliferation policy.

Patient care concerns manifest themselves in the labor field in two other ways. First, the rules on when and where union organizers can distribute union literature are particularly restrictive due to the concern for maintaining a tranquil hospital atmosphere. Generally, such solicitation activity is limited to nonworking hours and non-patient care areas of the hospital. *See* NLRB v. Baptist Hosp. Inc., 442 U.S. 773 (1979). Second, the NLRA requires a ten-day notice prior to striking or picketing a hospital, out of the obvious concern over avoiding disruption of care. 29 U.S.C. § 158(g). However, the NLRB and the courts have limited this requirement to authorized strikes of a recognized union, excluding wild-cat strikes by unrepresented employees.

b. Physician Unions

A question of labor law that will likely assume increasing importance over the next decade is whether physician unions are protected under the NLRA. In order to resist mounting institutional and economic pressures, doctors are beginning to form unions, particularly in the context of HMOs. However, limitations in the NLRA's coverage place substantial obstacles in their path. First, only employees have the right to unionize. This limitation has been used to exclude medical residents and interns from the protection of the Act under the theory that they are serving primarily as students, not employees. The limitation to employees would also seem to exclude independent physicians on a hospital medical staff from the NLRA's protections.

Second, even doctors who are employed may not be covered because the Act has long been interpreted to exclude "managerial employees" from its protections—those employees who assist management in determining and implementing policy. NLRB v. Bell Aerospace, 416 U.S. 267 (1974). This exclusion creates the prospect that employed physicians are never covered by the Act because health care institutions universally require heavy physician involvement on numerous committees that establish important medical policy. In a similar context, the Supreme Court determined (by a 5–4 vote) that the managerial employee exclusion applies to university professors because they participate on important committees and heavily influence faculty hiring decisions. NLRB v. Yeshiva University, 444 U.S. 672 (1980). However, the *Yeshiva* Court was wary of excluding all professional employees by this decision. Therefore, it cautioned that "employees whose decisionmaking is limited to the routine discharge of professional duties in projects to which they have been assigned cannot be excluded from coverage.... Only if an employee's activities fall outside the scope of the duties routinely performed by similarly situated professionals will he be found aligned with management." 444 U.S. at 690.

The NLRB has since wrestled with what this ruling might mean for the various administrative duties typically assigned to physicians within medical institutions, reaching conflicting results in its two principal decisions. In Montefiore Hospital, 261 N.L.R.B. 569 (1982), the Board distinguished *Yeshiva* in the context of employed physicians at a large teaching hospital, allowing them to form a union (even though, by coincidence, this hospital provided the teaching faculty for Yeshiva University's medical school!). The Board reasoned that, due to the highly structured hierarchical nature of the hospital's departmental organization, staff committees merely provided recommendations to departmental chairs and had no ultimate policymaking authority. In addition, the Board stressed that the staff's adoption of medical policy "does not necessarily fall outside the professional duties primarily incident to patient care." However, in FHP, Inc., 274 N.L.R.B.

1141 (1985), the Board followed *Yeshiva* and rejected a physician union at an HMO, giving an extensive rendition of the various committees on which
physicians served. The Board observed that "many
of the decisions made at the committee level ... lie
at the core of the [HMO's] operations" and that
"recommendations are regularly if not always followed." But, more recently, the Board reversed
course again and held that physicians at a different
HMO are not managerial and so can unionize.
Thomas–Davis Medical Centers, 324 NLRB No. 15
(1997).

Similar confusion reigns with respect to nurse
managers. In 1994, the Supreme Court ruled that
nurses employed in a nursing home exercised sufficient de facto supervision over the work assign-
ments of nurses' aides to be subject to the managerial exclusion. NLRB v. Health Care & Retirement
Corp. of America, 114 S.Ct. 1778 (1994). In a subsequent ruling, the NLRB refused to follow this precedent in a hospital setting, finding that hospital
"charge nurses" do not exercise the "independent
judgment" essential to finding supervisory status.
In yet another decision, the Board reached the same
result for a nursing home, finding that LPNs there
did not exercise supervisory authority over nursing
assistants.

It is difficult to reconcile these various decisions,
other than to observe that the inquiry is presently a
highly fact-sensitive one in which the particulars of
proof and the quality of lawyering makes a critical
difference. In reality, it is unlikely that there is a

tremendous difference between the authority of physician committees and nurse supervisors in these various settings. This unstable law results from the difficulty of adapting conventional notions of hierarchical corporate decisionmaking to the collegial environment of medical professionals.

2. Employment Law

a. *Wrongful Discharge*

In addition to the public regulatory law just surveyed, there have been important developments in private law doctrine that affect employment relationships in the health care sector. The most prominent development is the abrogation of the employment-at-will doctrine. Historically, employers have been free to fire workers with or without cause if they were hired without a specific contractual term of service. Over the last two decades, courts have so frequently found exceptions to this common law rule that some lawyers view the exceptions as having swallowed the rule. This doctrinal development is discussed here because, for some unknown reason, these employment-at-will disputes arise with surprising frequency in the health care industry.

There are three possible avenues for qualifying an at-will employer's freedom to fire. First, courts may find that the reason for firing an employee violates public policy, such as where an employer fires a "whistleblower" who reports safety violations to the proper authorities. See the discussion in section B.3 of HMO "deselection" suits. Second, employee manuals sometimes promise that procedural or substantive safeguards attach to the decision to terminate. If so, courts may find that these manual provisions have become implied-in-fact terms of the employment contract, under the reasoning that employees relied on these promised protections in deciding to stay on the job. Third, courts may rely on the covenant of good faith and fair dealing that the law implies into all contracts to hold that employers must give some good reason, and some fair process, when dismissing an employee, but this is only a minority position in the states.

Contrary to appearances, then, there has been no general abrogation of at-will employment in most jurisdictions; the exceptions to this rule remain just that. If employee manuals are carefully drafted, employers can avoid the contractual theory. As for the public policy theory, not every questionable reason for discharge violates public policy. Also, courts are careful to distinguish discharges based on behavior motivated by private concerns versus those motivated by public concerns. One situation, however, where health care employees are protected in their exercise of personal conscience is with respect to abortion. State and federal "conscience clause" statutes protect health care employees who refuse to perform abortions. 42 U.S.C. § 300a–7.

b. Covenants Not to Compete

A final area of importance in health care employment law arises from covenants not to compete in physician employment or managed care contracts.

In order to protect a practice group's interest in its established patients, physicians joining a group are usually required to abide by restrictive covenants that prevent them from practicing in the same geographic area for a certain period of time once they leave the group. However, courts view covenants not to compete in this and other employment contexts with suspicion because these restrictions contravene public policies in favor of free trade and the right to work. Restrictive covenants are valid only if they are reasonable as to time, geographic scope, and the range of activities covered, and if they are not otherwise contrary to the public interest. *See, e.g.,* Karpinski v. Ingrasci, 320 N.Y.S.2d 1 (1971) (restriction of defendant from practice of dentistry is overbroad where his employer practiced only oral surgery).

Of particular relevance in the medical context is whether it contravenes the public interest to restrain the practice of a physician whose services are needed in the community. For instance, in Dick v. Geist, 693 P.2d 1133 (Idaho App.1985), the court refused to enforce a restrictive covenant that would have excluded the two doctors who rendered 90% of the neonatal care in the community. Another line of cases has reasoned, though, that the public interest is equally well served even if the doctor is forced to treat patients in another part of the state.

CHAPTER 4

ANTITRUST LAW AND HEALTH CARE

A. INTRODUCTION

The federal antitrust laws have prompted one of
the most burgeoning areas of health care litigation
in recent years. Prior to 1980, antitrust challenges
to the health care industry were almost unheard of.
It was thought that the antitrust laws did not apply
to the learned professions and that health care is an
inherently local activity not subject to federal jurisdiction. The Supreme Court exploded both of these
myths in the mid 1970s. In Goldfarb v. Virginia
State Bar, 421 U.S. 773 (1975), a case concerning
the legal profession, the Court held that "the nature of an occupation, standing alone, does not
provide sanctuary from the Sherman Act." A year
later, the Court reinstated an antitrust suit against
a hospital, ruling that its operations have a substantial impact on interstate commerce by virtue of the
purchase of equipment and supplies and the receipt
of insurance reimbursement from out of state. Hospital Building Company v. Trustees of Rex Hospital,
425 U.S. 738 (1976).

The two-fisted blow of these decisions has left the
entire health care sector reeling ever since. Expo-

194

sure to antitrust scrutiny is a frightening prospect to doctors and hospitals because of the enormous potential liability. Damages awarded for lost business can be substantial and, under the antitrust laws, these damages are automatically tripled. Antitrust defendants may also have to pay for the costs of the plaintiff's attorneys if they lose. And, while most doctors and hospitals are well insured for malpractice, their insurance often does not cover antitrust liability. Finally, criminal enforcement actions can be brought by the government, possibly resulting in imprisonment.

This chapter explores four branches of health care antitrust law: group boycott challenges to a hospital's or HMO's exclusion of physicians from the medical staff; the price-fixing ramifications of health insurance and provider networks; vertical restraints and monopolization charges against HMOs; and merger doctrine as applied to various health care ventures.

B. ANTITRUST BOYCOTT LAW

Increasingly, medical staff disputes boil over into antitrust litigation, usually under section one of the Sherman Act, which prohibits conspiracies in restraint of interstate trade. 15 U.S.C. § 1. Physicians who are either denied admittance to the medical staff or whose staff privileges are revoked regularly characterize their exclusions as "concerted refusals to deal," or, more pejoratively, as group boycotts, which the Supreme Court has held from time to time in other contexts are per se illegal. Although antitrust law as a body is complex, this particular theory of action is rather straightforward: it is anticompetitive to allow physicians to exclude their competitors from hospital facilities that are essential for the practice of medicine.

1. The Conspiracy Requirement

In order for such a charge to be entertained under Sherman Act section one, the plaintiff must establish that a medical staff exclusion was the product of concerted (joint) rather than unilateral (single actor) behavior. This might seem to be a simple matter given the multiplicity of actors that usually participate in hospital credentialing decisions, but antitrust law generally looks to economic *entities* rather than individual *persons*. For example, it clearly does not constitute price fixing for the managers of a manufacturing firm to meet together to decide how to price their product, even though many people are involved in the decision, because they are all acting in the economic interest of a single entity—their employer. Such behavior does not present any anticompetitive threat because it does not "suddenly bring together economic power that was previously pursuing divergent goals." Copperweld Corp. v. Independence Tube Corp., 467 U.S. 752, 769 (1984). Likewise, in the context of medical staff membership decisions, it would initially appear that no conspiracy exists because physicians who participate in hospital peer review do so under the auspices of the hospital corporate entity.

However, there is an exception to this "intra-enterprise conspiracy" rule that is particularly problematic in this context. The rule applies only if those who claim its protection are pursuing a single economic interest—that of the hospital. Physicians, though, are not hospital employees; they have their own independent practices. Therefore, it is more than possible that a given physician might act out of the personal economic motive of not losing patients rather than out of concern for the quality of care at the hospital.

Most courts view the independent interest exception to the intra-enterprise conspiracy rule as a highly fact-sensitive judgment that inquires into the subjective motivations of the defendants. However, one early and influential decision, Weiss v. York Hospital, 745 F.2d 786 (3d Cir.1984), seemed to hold that all physicians who participate in peer review are engaged in a conspiracy *as a matter of law! Weiss* concerned the exclusion of an osteopath from a hospital medical staff controlled by M.D.s, and the court held that "the York medical staff is a group of doctors, all of whom practice medicine in their individual capacities, and each of whom is an independent economic entity in competition with other doctors in the York medical community."

There are two obvious difficulties with this analysis. First, it isn't true that all doctors have a competitive interest at stake with all other doctors. If Dr. Weiss (the physician who applied for privileges at York Hospital) had been a cardiac surgeon who limited his practice to pediatric patients, he might

have been in competition with very few doctors on
the medical staff. Even as a general practitioner, he
was not in competition with anesthesiologists, radiologists or pathologists. Second, even where potential for an independent, anticompetitive stake
exists, it would seem unfair to presume as a matter
of law that no physician is capable of setting that
interest aside and acting solely out of the hospital's
concern for quality of care. Therefore, other decisions have allowed factual presentations on these
issues, but that hardly constitutes a safe harbor.
Accordingly, the safest alternative is to structure
the peer review process so that only non-competing
doctors are involved, even if this means delegating
review functions to doctors who live elsewhere.
Medical staffs typically are unwilling to relinquish
this control, however.

2. Medical Staff Boycotts as Restraints of Trade

a. Avoiding Per Se Illegality

A Sherman Act section one plaintiff, if she clears
the conspiracy hurdle, must next establish that the
challenged behavior constitutes a restraint of trade.
The courts have made a broad division between two
types of tests to judge the multitude of economic
behavior that potentially constitutes a restraint of
trade. If a given practice is so obviously anticompetitive that it can virtually never be justified—for
example, price fixing among competitors—the
courts apply the "per se illegal" label and find an
antitrust violation as a matter of law. All other

challenged business activity is judged under some version of the rule of reason, which seeks to balance the activity's anticompetitive effects against its pro-competitive effects.

This reasonableness inquiry traditionally has required a lengthy trial with a host of economic and industry experts. Therefore, even this lesser standard of liability gives the physician-plaintiff strong leverage for bargaining since hospitals will find it difficult to prevail at a summary judgment stage under this fact-sensitive analysis. However, in recent years the federal courts have begun to use more lenient forms of the rule of reason that demand a greater showing of the plaintiff in order to survive the defendant's motion for summary judgment. *Cf.* Matsushita Electric Indus. Co. v. Zenith Radio Corp., 475 U.S. 574 (1986).

Group boycotts, otherwise known as "concerted refusals to deal," constitute one category of activity that has received the per se label. In the paradigm case, a group of retailers refuses to deal with a wholesaler who is cooperating with another retailer outside of the group. But "group boycott" is simply a pejorative label that might attach to any concerted refusal to associate with someone else, and one can think of any number of such actions that are socially beneficial, such as where a professional society excludes a member for engaging in unethical behavior. Therefore, a great deal of controversy surrounds the general question in antitrust theory of which group boycotts are automatically per se illegal.

In the context of hospital peer review, Weiss v. York Hospital, 745 F.2d 786 (3d Cir.1984), is again instructive. There, the court wrestled with fitting a medical staff exclusion decision into the classic boycott mold. A hospital might be viewed in the chain of production of medical services as equivalent to a wholesaler, and doctors might be viewed as retailers. Therefore, to match the paradigm case, doctors would have to exclude a competitor by threatening to leave the hospital. This could be called a "secondary boycott" because it is directed at one party (the hospital) in order to reach a second (the competing physician). Doctors have little reason to engage in the classic paradigm of a secondary boycott, however, since they have the ability to engage directly in a *primary* boycott of an unwanted competitor. Existing medical staff members, because of their influence over credentialing decisions, can exclude a competitor simply by deciding themselves not to deal with a medical staff applicant rather than attempting to coerce the hospital not to deal with the competitor.

The *Weiss* court found this incongruity in paradigms much more troubling than it actually is. Primary boycotts are rare in antitrust precedents only because few industries are structured like the medical profession to allow existing competitors to expel or block the entry of potential competitors. The per se illegality of primary boycotts follows *a fortiori* from the precedents that address secondary boycotts.

Thus, there are strong precedential and theoretical grounds to be wary of medical staff exclusions. On the other hand, the role of physician peer review is vital to maintaining the safety of medical treatment. State medical licensure boards (like state bars) do little to ensure the continuing competence of practitioners, so the critical weeding-out task falls on hospitals, who must necessarily delegate the decision to those with knowledge and expertise— their member physicians. Moreover, it is through the peer review process that hospitals compete among themselves on the basis of their quality of care by attempting to select the very best doctors available. To essentially outlaw medical peer review therefore would have disastrous consequences.

Medical peer review thus confronts antitrust analysis with a unique paradox: heightened anti-competitive risk coupled with heightened social need. As a result, this is not an area that lends itself well to the traditional dichotomy offered by the sharp doctrinal distinction between the rule of reason and per se illegality. What one would like to do is to take a quick look at each case to see if legitimate reasons have been advanced for adverse action against a medical professional. If so, then the rule of reason would be appropriate. If not, then the per se rule should be applied.

This bifurcated analysis appears to reflect the dominant approach that the courts have in fact taken in medical staff cases. In Weiss v. York Hospital, *supra*, for instance, the jury found that Dr. Weiss had been excluded as a result of the medical staff's bias against osteopaths generally and the defendants did not attempt to advance a legitimate (*i.e.*, quality-of-care based) justification for their discriminatory action. Consequently, the court applied the per se label. However, the court stated that had the hospital excluded osteopaths "on the basis of their lack of professional competence or unprofessional conduct, ... the rule of reason, rather than a per se rule, would be applicable."

This ruling appears to comport with the Supreme Court's subsequent decision in Northwest Wholesale Stationers Inc. v. Pacific Stationery and Printing Co., 472 U.S. 284, 294 (1985). There, the Court explained in another context that "the mere allegation of a concerted refusal to deal does not suffice because not all concerted refusals to deal are predominantly anticompetitive." Therefore, "a plaintiff seeking application of the *per se* rule must present a threshold case that the challenged activity falls into a category likely to have predominantly anticompetitive effects." The Court noted that, in cases where this showing has been made in the past, the challenged practices "generally were not justified by plausible arguments that they were intended to enhance overall efficiency and make markets more competitive."

The York Hospital medical staff's failure to articulate a quality-of-care justification for a medical staff membership policy is rare in antitrust litigation. Virtually every other case has been decided under a rule of reason analysis because most hospitals readily establish at least the pretext of a quality justification. For example, in F.T.C. v. Indiana Federation of Dentists, 476 U.S. 447 (1986), the Court applied the rule of reason to a professional dentist society's refusal to submit dental X-rays to insurance companies, even though this is ordinarily a per se illegal group boycott, because the dentists justified this practice based on the quality-of-care rationale that X-rays alone are an insufficient basis on which to determine the medical necessity for dental services.

b. Avoiding Trial on the Merits

It is fairly easy for antitrust defenders to make the necessary allegations to avoid per se condemnation of medical staff decisions, but that is only the first line of defense in these cases. Defense attorneys are also eager to avoid trial on the merits, both because this is so time-consuming and expensive, and also because individual physicians denied the chance to practice their profession are sympathetic figures in jury trials. Courts too are reluctant to let these cases go to trial out of the judicial instinct that they are nothing more than individual personnel disputes, which should not be turned into federal antitrust cases.

This instinct has expressed itself in a number of different areas of doctrine that allow courts to render summary judgment for the defense, despite plausible assertions of anticompetitive conduct by excluded physicians. Most of these rulings rely on the notion that antitrust law protects competition rather than competitors. This slogan reflects the idea that, even though the economic harm to an individual physician may be great, competition itself is not harmed as long as there are plenty of other physicians around to pick up the slack. Thus, courts are inclined to dismiss these cases outright if the remaining physicians do not exercise significant market power. Even when courts allow these cases to go to trial, they frequently exert a very lenient level of scrutiny, one that asks only whether the hospital had a rational basis and some evidentiary support for the exclusion, and not whether, on the merits, the court thinks the charges against the physician are true. As advocated by Professor Clark Havighurst, the leading commentator on health care antitrust:

> To ensure that hospitals have reasonable freedom of action, ... summary judgment or a directed verdict would be appropriate if documentary evidence and affidavits showed that the hospital's action reflected its [own] corporate concerns.... Under this test, a court would not concern itself ... with whether the ostensible motives for the actions taken were the real motives or whether the adverse effect of the hospital action on competition among practitioners was outweighed by its actual contribution to fulfilling the hospital's objectives.

Clark Havighurst, Doctors and Hospitals: An Antitrust Perspective on Traditional Relationships, 1984 Duke L.J. 1071, 1133–34, 1157.

Courts are most likely to follow this course when adverse action is taken against a single physician based on his individual competence, rather than in a case that excludes an entire class of practitioners or that is clearly motivated by economic rivalry. The same attitude is captured in the qualified immunity statute discussed in chapter 4.C.6.b, which applies only to individual physician exclusions based on quality, and not to group-based exclusions, exclusions of non-physicians, or those based on economic grounds.

3. Exclusions From Managed Care Networks and Illegal Tie-ins

This same body of law potentially applies as well to the exclusion of physicians from managed care networks. One of the leading cases serves well to illustrate how the principles above apply in this slightly different context. In Hassan v. Independent Practice Associates, 698 F. Supp. 679 (E.D.Mich. 1988), an HMO removed from its network two allergists whom it thought were ordering too many tests. First, the court found there was a potential conspiracy since primary care physicians were involved in the decision and they compete for some of the same business. Next, however, the court declined to apply the per se rule of illegality. Even though no quality of care issues were raised, the economic issues advanced by the HMO appeared legitimate. When it came to examining the merits, however, the court ruled on summary judgment in favor of the HMO. It observed that the HMO had little market power since the HMO controlled only 20 percent of the insurance market, and the allergists were free to contract with other plans. Also, the other physicians had nonexclusive contracts with the HMO which made it easier for new HMOs to enter the market. Finally, the HMO subsequently admitted two other allergists to the network, which contradicted the claim that primary care physicians were trying to take over the allergy business.

One way plaintiffs might respond to these arguments is that HMO market power is potentially much stronger if viewed more narrowly, by looking at the set of patients who are current subscribers. For them, a physician's exclusion from the network has dramatic effect because, as long as they are members, they cannot shop for care from excluded physicians. For this set of patients, the HMO has 100 percent market share, and options within the network are limited. This analysis resonates with Eastman Kodak v. Image Technical Services, 504 U.S. 451 (1992), in which the Court held that a separate submarket could exist for the parts required to repair a Kodak brand photocopy machine if Kodak parts are not interchangeable with parts from other brands, since once someone purchases the expensive machine, they are locked in to buying only Kodak parts. This is similar to another theory of antitrust injury known as an illegal tie-in, which has also been declared to be per se illegal. A tie-in exists when a firm with market power over one product insists that purchasers also pay for another product they don't necessarily want.

Whether this line of analysis is convincing is subject to debate. HMOs do have a lock-in, but not for life, only for potentially a year, and perhaps much shorter. Moreover, the lock-in is often not absolute, since many plans now allow patients to go outside the network by paying a somewhat higher copay or deductible. As for the tie-in characterization, the Court surprisingly accepted this characterization in a case in which a hospital required surgery patients to use only the anesthesiologists it had under exclusive contract. However, the Court found no violation since the particular hospital lacked the requisite market power to coerce the patient's choice of an anesthesiologist. Jefferson Parish Hospital District v. Hyde, 466 U.S. 2 (1984).

At the moment, then, it appears that HMOs have fairly free reign to pick and drop their network providers as they see fit. Whether courts would be as lenient with hospitals for their economic-based exclusions is another matter. One is used to condemning hospital exclusions if they are based on the economic motives of member *physicians,* but in today's market environment, hospitals have their *own* economic interests to protect, and these, in contrast with member physicians' economic interests, are a legitimate basis for an institutional decision. After all, hospitals' quality interest is, at bottom, economic in nature, at least in the antitrust mindset, since maintaining quality enhances one's reputation in the market and reduces malpractice liability.

4. The Patient Care Defense

Some medical staff exclusion cases do receive close antitrust scrutiny because, even though the stated reasons for exclusion might be legitimate enough to avoid per se condemnation, since there is enough potential for anticompetitive harm to warrant fact-based rule of reason balancing. For hospitals and professional associations, the critical issue then becomes precisely how quality of care concerns are incorporated into what normally is a purely economic inquiry into the procompetitive versus anticompetitive effects of a refusal to deal.

For a time, it was thought that all of the learned professions might impliedly be exempt from the antitrust laws because of the influence of professional ethics and public service norms on their behavior. But in Goldfarb v. Virginia State Bar, 421 U.S. 773 (1975), a case concerning lawyers' fee schedules, the Supreme Court rejected any such sweeping exemption. However, the Court left behind some pregnant dictum whose meaning still has not been fully articulated: "the public service aspect, and other features of the professions, may require that a particular practice, which could properly be viewed as a violation of the Sherman Act in another context, be treated differently." 421 U.S. at 778 n. 17.

One effect of this dictum appears to be that conduct otherwise falling within the per se prohibition will be judged under the rule of reason if the conduct is "premised on public service or ethical norms." Arizona v. Maricopa County Medical Society, 457 U.S. 332, 348–49 (1982). But this merely restates the analysis above. It does not address the additional question of, assuming that the rule of reason applies, exactly how the rule takes account of these norms. At first, it was thought that the effect of the *Goldfarb* dictum would be to apply a sort of "relaxed" rule of reason analysis to the professions, one that gives heavy deference to judgments concerning the demands of public safety. However, the Court squarely rejected any such special approach for safety concerns in National Society of Professional Engineers v. United States, 435 U.S. 679 (1978). There, the Court held that the rule of reason "does not open the field of antitrust inquiry to any argument in favor of a challenged restraint that may fall within the realm of reason. ... [T]he inquiry is confined to a consideration of impact on competitive conditions."

This might appear to place hospitals and doctors in an intolerable dilemma: tort law forces them to review the competence of medical staff members, but antitrust law's refusal to entertain non-economic justifications for physician exclusions appears to exclude any quality-of-care defense. This appearance is deceiving, however. It is patently wrong to conceive of economic motives and quality of care as mutually opposed considerations in hospital staffing decisions. Indeed, from the hospital's perspective, the two are *co*extensive because *quality is the key competitive variable in the hospital industry*. Indeed, for decades quality competition was virtually the sole force that drove the entire health care sector. Therefore, quality of care concerns factor directly into the procompetitive side of the rule of reason balance.

A good illustration of how this outline analysis might apply in an actual case comes from Wilk v. American Medical Association, 671 F.Supp. 1465 (N.D.Ill.1987), which addresses the AMA's long-standing opposition to the chiropractic profession. Although this case does not concern a medical staff exclusion, it reflects another body of caselaw that addresses rules set by professional societies. The district court found that the AMA's refusal to allow physicians to associate with chiropractors consti-tutes an unreasonable restraint of trade. In doing so, however, the court, following an earlier 7th Circuit opinion in the same case, allowed the AMA to assert an affirmative defense based on its con-cerns over the unscientific nature of chiropractic. This defense required the AMA to show that its concern was objectively reasonable and that it could not have been satisfied in less restrictive means than a total boycott. The court ruled that the AMA satisfied the first element but not the second.

Although *Wilk* reached the correct outcome, its reasoning has been criticized for misconstruing how quality of care concerns should be considered in more typical cases. Consider, for instance, a hospital that decides to exclude chiropractors. It seems ex-cessive to place the burden of proof on the hospital to prove they are dangerous to patients. On the other hand, in the *Wilk* case, it appears inconsistent

with Supreme Court precedent to potentially allow
the AMA off the hook for its good motives if in fact
the blatant boycott was anticompetitive. How does
one resolve these conflicting impressions? The key
is to distinguish between an ordinary defense and
an affirmative defense. Where quality is legitimately
a competitive factor for a single entity, as it is for a
hospital but not for the AMA (which is a walking
conspiracy), then quality of care should be considered as a direct or ordinary defense. An ordinary
defense leaves the burden of proof on the plaintiff
and requires only a showing that the decision improved quality to some degree, not that it was
necessary to avoid incompetence in any absolute
sense. In this situation, an affirmative defense is
unnecessary, and its proof standards are too demanding. However, where quality is not a legitimate competitive factor, then there is no justification for constructing a special defense that forgives
antitrust violators because of their good intentions.

5. The Interstate Commerce and State Action Defenses

Two other defenses deserve brief mention. For a
time some courts rejected federal antitrust challenges to medical disputes because they viewed
medical care as an inherently local matter that does
not constitute interstate commerce. However, the
Supreme Court has clarified that there is sufficient
impact on interstate commerce to invoke federal
jurisdiction because medical care uses supplies from
out of state and is often paid for by out-of-state

insurers. Summit Health v. Pinhas, 500 U.S. 322 (1991).

A few other courts also rejected these challenges under a more obscure defense known as "state action immunity," which reasons that Congress never intended to apply antitrust law to state government. For instance, it would be spurious to charge a state Board of Medical Examiners with an antitrust violation for revoking a physician's license. The state action defense potentially exists with respect to physician discipline even at *private* hospitals if state law mandates and "actively supervises" the private peer review process. The Court rejected this contention, however, in Patrick v. Burget, 486 U.S. 94 (1988), holding that private hospital credentialing decisions in Oregon are not sufficiently supervised by the state to bring them within the protection of this defense. The court observed that Oregon, unlike other states, had not yet recognized a common law right of judicial review of credentialing decisions.

Although *Patrick* was initially read as closing the door to state action immunity, it left open the small crack of a possibility that immunity might exist in another state whose common law differs. However, it is unlikely that any common law theory of judicial review would meet the Court's objection that "the review [is] of a very limited nature ... [in which the courts do no] more than make sure that some sort of reasonable procedure was afforded and that there was evidence from which it could be found that plaintiff's conduct posed a threat to patient care." On the other hand, a state might, if it chose to, impose this type of supervision through regulatory rather than judicial channels. A number of states have done so in the form of "certificate of public advantage" (CPA) laws, which set up an explicit system for giving state regulatory blessing to cooperative agreements that are viewed as beneficial to the community but which might otherwise violate the antitrust laws. This state review process is designed to meet the active supervision requirement. For the most part, however, these statutes do not apply to peer review decisions. Instead, they are directed to joint ventures and mergers, like those discussed below, in which hospitals and other providers seek to cooperate in order to achieve efficiencies and avoid costly duplication of facilities.

C. PRICE FIXING AND VERTICAL RESTRAINTS INVOLVING INSURERS

1. Price Fixing in Provider Networks

The primary example of per se illegality is horizontal price fixing, defined as any agreement among horizontal competitors (*i.e.*, firms at the same level within the marketplace) concerning the price or quality of their products, usually, an agreement not to undercut each others' price. The per se illegality of price fixing presents a danger in the establishment of various innovative forms of health insurance. The clearest example comes from preferred provider organizations (PPOs), but this analysis applies to other types of provider networks that enter into managed care arrangements. PPOs are groups of health care providers that agree to sell their services at a discount in exchange for receiving a large supply of business, say, all the employees covered by a large group insurance policy. PPOs are sometimes initiated by insurance companies or employers, who contact health care providers individually and negotiate discounts one by one. Such "consumer-based" PPOs raise no price fixing concern because the consumer group establishes a separate bilateral contract with each provider. More typically, though, PPOs are initiated by doctors or hospitals who approach consumer groups and offer their discounted terms in a united fashion. (Perhaps this is more common because of the lower transaction costs involved in this form of contract negotiation.) Provider-based PPOs must be organized as *groups* of doctors because no one physician could provide the bulk services required by a large insurance group. However, such "provider-based PPOs," and other kinds of provider networks, raise the distinct aura of price fixing since all of the doctors or hospitals first agree among themselves what price to charge or what discount to give to employers or insurers.

The price-fixing potential of provider-based PPOs was confirmed by the Supreme Court in Arizona v. Maricopa County Medical Society, 457 U.S. 332 (1982). Although *Maricopa County* did not address a PPO in name, the health care delivery plan at issue there (called a "foundation for medical care") was structurally identical to a PPO. The medical society in Maricopa County (Phoenix) sponsored a plan whereby all participating physicians agreed to abide by a maximum fee schedule if insurers agreed to pay 100% of those fees. Almost three quarters of the physicians in the county were members. The Court ruled that this arrangement constituted per se illegal price fixing. The Court was not concerned that the agreement set a cap on fees rather than a floor, since either could equally well serve as a benchmark for uniform pricing behavior, and, in any event, a cap on fees reduces *quality* competition if not *price* competition.

Maricopa County was decided by a 4–3 plurality vote as the result of two Justices abstaining. This fact, coupled with the subsequent change in Court members, raises the possibility that a majority of the Court would reach a different result if confronted with this issue again, or would limit this holding strictly to its facts. The frailty of the *Maricopa County* holding is highlighted by a set of antitrust enforcement guidelines issued jointly by the Department of Justice Antitrust Division and the FTC. These guidelines do not directly alter the law, but they do state when these agencies will exercise their enforcement discretion to challenge provider-based PPOs and other contracting networks. The DOJ/ FTC guidelines in essence judge PPOs under a rule of reason rather than a per se analysis. They express concern only if the arrangement involves a large percentage of the area's providers or if there is an overt indication of anticompetitive intent. The enforcement guidelines also establish several safe harbors that protect provider networks from any significant agency scrutiny. Therefore, despite the fact that *Maricopa County* still expresses established law, it is possible for thoughtful health care lawyers to devise several ways to sidestep the four corners of the *Maricopa County* holding by fine tuning the structure of provider-based PPOs to avoid application of the ominous price fixing characterization.

The cleanest way to avoid a horizontal price-fixing charge is to realign the agreement from a horizontal to a vertical dimension. This most clearly happens if the purchaser (insurer or employer) determines the price it is willing to pay and lets each doctor decide unilaterally whether or not to join. Although this appears to produce exactly the same result—a group of doctors agreeing on the same payment terms with one or more purchasers—the absence of a horizontal agreement among physicians removes this from per se price fixing.

The trouble is that physicians often want to take the initiative in forming these network arrangements, for both strategic and efficiency reasons. To allow this to continue, crafty health care lawyers have devised a way to dress a horizontal arrangement in vertical clothing, known as the "messenger model." In this arrangement, physicians agree to use a common negotiating agent to establish bilateral price agreements with purchasers. In the cleanest version, the agent conveys to each physician the insurer's price, and each physician decides whether to opt in. The DOJ/FTC guidelines approve this opt in version of the messenger model. Much more suspect, however, is a "black box" or "opt out" version in which physicians agree in advance to be bound by whatever payment terms the agent is able to negotiate, unless they opt out. Although physicians do not strictly speaking agree in advance to fixed price terms, their pricing is sufficiently coordinated that the effect is virtually the same, so the enforcement guidelines prohibit this approach. Other inventive messenger approaches that fall between these two versions are also possible but have not been clearly ruled on.

A second technique for avoiding the *Maricopa County* holding is for the participating physicians, rather than merely establishing a loose contractual relationship, to integrate into a single economic entity by forming, say, a large partnership in which they pool their assets and share business risks. Here again, inventive lawyering has found several ways to accomplish the substance or appearance of business integration without having to resort to the full scale version. The economic substance of integration can be achieved by exposing physicians to shared financial risk. The *Maricopa County* decision itself says this occurs if physicians accept capitation payment. The DOJ/FTC guidelines also mention fee withholds and other risk-based payment methods. The unresolved issues here are how extensive the financial risk must be, and whether the risk-based payments must cover all physician services or only some (primary care capitation versus global capitation). Note also that encouraging physicians to accept capitation payment to avoid antitrust risk conflicts with other legal signals discussed elsewhere, which discourage risk-based payment either by prohibiting or limiting financial conflicts of interest or by treating risk-bearing providers as if they were insurance companies.

A third possible way to avoid the *Maricopa County* holding is to create some new product. This avenue is suggested by the controversial and difficult case of Broadcast Music, Inc. v. Columbia Broadcasting System, Inc., 441 U.S. 1 (1979), where the Court held that the bulk licensing of music compositions does not constitute per se price fixing even though competing composers necessarily agree among themselves how much to charge for their songs. The Court reasoned in *BMI*, that this arrangement in effect creates a new product—a "blanket license" for all BMI compositions, and price-setting is merely ancillary to this procompetitive device. Likewise, it might be contended that the bulk sale of medical services through a physician network creates a new product, particularly since networks usually offer a package of related services such as claims processing and utilization review. However, in *Maricopa County*, the Court distinguished *BMI* by holding in essence that these additional services amount to nothing more than window dressing and that PPOs do not offer a new and distinct health care product. The Court suggested that an HMO would meet this new product test, but this is simply another way of restating the financial integration defense just summarized. The DOJ/FTC guidelines take a more lenient view, however, by holding out the possibility of avoiding per se condemnation by showing *clinical* integration. It is unclear what exactly clinical integration means, other than actual group practices in the same clinical setting, but the guidelines suggest the very same elements of peer review and common clinical protocols that were found insufficient in *Maricopa County*. The enforcement agencies have yet to rule on very many such cases, however, so we don't know how easily imaginative lawyers and managers will be able to devise arrangements that will meet the requirements for a *BMI*-type defense.

A word of caution: most of what has been said in this section applies only to *physician*, not hospital, networks. Hospital networks raise much more serious antitrust concerns since there are far fewer hospitals than doctors in any given market and so the dangers of collaboration are much greater.

2. Monopolization by Insurers

More conventional insurance practices have also been subject to antitrust attack. Most cases concern insurers either limiting the amount that physicians can bill or excluding certain categories of health care providers. In one leading case, Blue Shield was sued unsuccessfully for imposing a ban on "balance billing," that is, prohibiting participating physicians from charging patients any more than the contractual amount paid by the insurance policy. Kartell v. Blue Shield of Massachusetts, 749 F.2d 922 (1st

Cir.1984). In a second leading case, Blue Cross was sued successfully for limiting coverage of mental health services from clinical psychologists that were fully covered when rendered by psychiatrists. Virginia Academy of Clinical Psychologists v. Blue Shield, 624 F.2d 476 (4th Cir.1980). How can these two cases be reconciled?

Restrictive reimbursement policies are clearly valid under Sherman Act section one if they are imposed unilaterally by a single insurance company. This is a vertical, not a horizontal restraint, in which a purchaser simply declares how much it is willing to pay. Even monopolistic purchasers may do this. However, the historical fact that Blue Cross and Blue Shield are creatures of the hospital industry and the medical profession (respectively) suggests that it is sometimes possible to establish that insurance restrictions are the result of collaboration among providers. For example, in Reazin v. Blue Cross & Blue Shield of Kansas, 899 F.2d 951 (10th Cir.1990), the court sustained a $7.8 million jury verdict against Blue Cross for conspiring with one local hospital to exclude another from a PPO arrangement. In *Virginia Academy supra*, the court held that the mere fact that physicians controlled the board of Blue Shield was sufficient to bring that company's unilateral actions under the purview of Sherman Act section one. However, most Blues plans have reconstituted their boards so that they are not dominated by physicians or hospitals. Consequently, it is now more difficult to show the existence of a horizontal conspiracy behind the actions of a single insurer and so more recent decisions have refused to entertain a section one theory.

Nevertheless, insurance restrictions may be challenged under Sherman Act section two, which prohibits unilateral monopolization or attempts to monopolize. The elements of these theories are not easy to meet, however. Monopolization requires a showing of a dominant market share and the use of illicit business practices. Attempted monopolization requires a showing of specific intent to monopolize and a likelihood of success. Most section two attacks have failed to meet these requirements. *See, e.g., Kartell supra* (no section two violation in limiting amount doctors can charge, despite 74% market share); Ball Memorial Hosp. v. Mutual Hosp. Ins. Inc., 784 F.2d 1325 (7th Cir.1986) (no monopoly despite 50–80% market share).

Particular insurer practices have come under scrutiny recently, however. One is requiring that providers contract with a dominant insurer on an exclusive basis. This makes it very difficult for new insurers to enter the market, since existing providers have to give up their existing business to sign on with the new insurer. Therefore, the enforcement agencies and several court opinions look with disfavor on these exclusive provider contracts. One might respond that mutually exclusive competing provider networks are a superior market configuration than nonexclusive overlapping provider networks because this makes each insurers' product more distinct and it allows insurers to impose more market discipline on providers by forcing them to engage in competitive bidding for network slots. These competitive benefits have to be weighed against the competitive harms of exclusive contracts, however, and most analysts believe that such contracts are dangerous in highly concentrated insurance or provider markets.

A related insurer technique is known as a "most favored nation" provision. In this technique, an existing dominant insurer (say, Blue Cross) tells its providers that they must give it the same payment discounts they agree to give any other insurer. This makes it very difficult for new insurers to enter the market by undercutting the dominant insurers' reimbursement rates, since any provider who agrees to the discounted rate for a small portion of their patients must then give the same discount for all their patients. Nevertheless, courts so far have upheld most favored nation provisions, reasoning that they are simply a way of requiring providers to make their best price available to everyone. In the words of one court, "this, it would seem, is what competition should be all about." Ocean State Physicians Health Plan v. Blue Cross & Blue Shield of Rhode Island, 883 F.2d 1101 (1st Cir. 1989). Others, including the enforcement agencies, view this thinking as naive, especially in markets where an insurer has a dominant share, since this is simply another way to make market entry or expansion more difficult for potential competitors, similar to the use of exclusive contracts.

3. McCarran–Ferguson Exemption

Before leaving the arena of insurance and anti-trust, it is necessary to observe briefly that insurance companies have a potential defense under the McCarran–Ferguson Act, 15 U.S.C. § 1011, which exempts the business of insurance from antitrust and other federal laws. Although this exemption appears sweeping, the Supreme Court has construed it very narrowly to apply only to those specific activities that are at the very core of insurance's risk-spreading function and that implicate the direct relationship between insurers and subscribers. *See* chapter 5.C. Thus, the exemption does not apply to insurers' contracts or dealings with providers, since this is ancillary to or behind the scenes of the main insurance contract. Group Life & Health Insurance Co. v. Royal Drug Co., 440 U.S. 205 (1979).

D. MERGER LAW

Section seven of the Clayton Act prohibits mergers that "substantially lessen competition or tend to create a monopoly." 15 U.S.C. § 18. The principal concern of this prohibition is to keep markets from becoming so concentrated in a few large firms that it becomes easy for the major firms to collude. The legality of mergers is usually assessed under certain numerical tests that focus on the size and the number of firms and their market shares before and after a merger. Market share definition is also critical to other antitrust theories, so much of this discussion is relevant throughout this chapter.

One leading hospital merger case is Hospital Corporation of America (HCA) v. Federal Trade Commission (FTC), 807 F.2d 1381 (7th Cir.1986), where Judge Posner wrote the opinion sustaining an FTC decision that prohibited the country's largest hospital chain from acquiring several hospitals in the Chattanooga market. Prior to the acquisition, HCA owned only one hospital in the market. Afterwards, it owned or managed 5 of the 11 area hospitals. This acquisition resulted in four firms controlling 91 percent of the market. The court reasoned that this degree of market concentration is dangerous given the history of cooperation between competing hospitals in Chattanooga and the barrier that CON regulation creates to new hospitals entering the market.

Hospitals are not the only object of merger analysis in health care. Physician groups and managed care networks are also subject to merger scrutiny. The DOJ/FTC guidelines set safe harbor protections that allow only 20–30 percent of the physicians in any given specialty to form a network without requiring agency approval. (The higher threshold applies only if physicians contract on a nonexclusive basis.) Similarly, a hospital's joint venture with its medical staff, for instance to operate an ambulatory surgery clinic, might be the subject of a merger challenge.

Because market share statistics control merger analysis, merger cases are often won or lost based on how the relevant market is defined. Ordinarily, the larger the market, the less significant will be the challenged firm's acquisition. There are two dimensions to the determination of market size: the geographic market and the product market. In the *HCA* case, for instance, the FTC used as the geographic market an area comprising the counties that are commonly recognized as encompassing the Chattanooga metropolitan area; the FTC rejected the contention that outlying rural counties should be included even though some patients from those counties may occasionally travel into Chattanooga for highly specialized care. Other courts, however, have been convinced to accept geographic markets encompassing a dozen or so counties surrounding a metropolitan area, reasoning that, if prices increase too much, people will be willing to travel to receive care. One court observed that, even if this was not the case earlier, it is now very much the reality for HMO patients, since HMOs regularly force people to bypass nearby hospitals in order to use ones that the HMO contracts with. FTC v. Freeman Hospital, 69 F.3d 260 (8th Cir.1995).

The other dimension of market definition is to define the relevant product. In *HCA*, the FTC looked solely at the operations of general hospitals. Thus, it excluded specialty hospitals that render only psychiatric care even though some general hospitals also treat psychiatric patients, but it included *all* the operations of general hospitals, both their inpatient business and their outpatient business, despite the fact that many nonhospital institutions also render similar outpatient care. These

findings are recited not as stating binding precedent—for such determinations are highly fact-spe-
cific and thus are subject to proof in each case—but
instead are given to illustrate the complexity of
analysis that is required to determine whether a
proposed merger creates an antitrust risk.

Consider also what the proper product market
definition is in cases involving HMOs. In Blue Cross
& Blue Shield United of Wisconsin v. Marshfield
Clinic, 65 F.3d 1406 (7th Cir. 1995), another opinion
by Judge Posner overturned a plaintiff's jury ver-
dict based on a ruling that HMOs are not a separate
market since they compete with indemnity insurers.
This suggests markets for insurance whose scope is
statewide or perhaps even national, since the leading indemnity insurers compete nationally. The
Marshfield case also discusses what the proper
product scope is for physician markets. The court
rejected the plaintiffs' allegation that physician services should be broken into markets for each specific service by DRG category depending on how many
physicians are currently performing each procedure.
The court observed that most medical services can
be performed by physicians in several different spe-
cialties so that if a given procedure were being
monopolized there are always plenty of other physicians ready to compete. Therefore, Judge Posner
appeared to use a market definition encompassing
all physicians. The DOJ/FTC guidelines, in contrast,
require that physician services be evaluated by specialty. They do not define, however, what consti-

tutes a specialty. Consider, for instance, whether
pediatric cardiac surgery constitutes a unique market or instead falls within the broader categories of
surgery or cardiac surgery.

Although market share statistics dominate merger analysis, they are not the sole determinants of
legality. Even mergers that monopolize a market
may potentially pass muster: (1) if the acquired
firm would have failed but for the merger; (2) if the
market is too small to support more than one or a
few hospitals (which is called a "natural monopoly"); or (3) if there are other factors that indicate
the merger is beneficial to the public. For instance,
the DOJ/FTC guidelines create a safe harbor for
mergers involving hospitals with fewer than 100
beds and 40 patients a day, even if the merger
results in only one hospital remaining in the market. Other courts have allowed hospital mergers to
go forward in highly concentrated markets because
of the offsetting concentration of buying power in
insurers. In FTC v. Butterworth Health Corp., 946
F.Supp. 1285 (W.D.Mich.1996), *aff'd*, 121 F.3d 708
(6th Cir. 1997), the court reversed the FTC and
permitted the merger of the two dominant hospitals
in Grand Rapids, Michigan, observing that financially sound hospitals are necessary to counteract
the growing threat of HMOs and "to continue the
quest for establishment of world-class health facilities in West Michigan." In *HCA* supra, however, the
court rejected a similar contention with respect to
the buying power of Blue Cross.

A final area of controversy is whether the non-profit status of most hospitals alters the nature of merger (or other antitrust) analysis. There are two distinct issues. One is whether, as a technical jurisdictional matter, the Clayton Act applies at all to nonprofit institutions. This question has been resolved in the affirmative. FTC v. University Health, 938 F.2d 1206 (11th Cir. 1991). The second question is whether nevertheless there is less concern about mergers among nonprofits, following the logic that nonprofits are less interested in profiteering by taking advantage of market power. Some cynics, such as Judge Posner in the *HCA* case and his other opinions, think nonprofits have essentially the same motive as for-profits to make as much money as possible. The only difference is what nonprofits can do with the money they make. Others, however, like *Butterworth* supra, believe that nonprofits are more likely to act cooperatively in a fashion that benefits the community at large by reducing excess capacity and improving coordination of services, following the health planning tradition reflected in the CON laws. This debate is informed to some extent by conflicting empirical findings, some of which show that mergers among nonprofit hospitals, even in highly concentrated markets, lead to reduced costs and prices, but others showing the contrary.

Each of these contested issues reveals that courts are taking an active role in setting antitrust policy for the health care industry. By doing so, courts are being much less deferential to the FTC and DOJ than they typically are in antitrust matters. There are increasing signs of judicial annoyance at treating health care just like any other industry, and increasing insistence that the enforcement agencies recognize the unique attributes of health insurance and medical care rather than rely on general economic theories.

CHAPTER 5

COMPLEX TRANSACTIONS AND ORGANIZATIONAL FORMS

As a consequence of increasing regulation and rapidly changing economic and legal forces, hospitals, doctors, and insurance companies are forming all manner of new organizational approaches to health care delivery and insurance, resulting in an explosion of acronyms. In the 1970s, we saw the birth of Health Maintenance Organizations (HMOs), a form of prepaid group medical practice explored in chapter 1.A.2.f. This was followed in the 1980s by the creation of Preferred Provider Organizations (PPOs), a form of bulk purchase of medical services explored in chapter 4.C.1. These are only the principal examples of new integrated delivery systems ("IDSs"). Physicians and hospitals are forming joint venture organizations (called PHOs for physician-hospital organizations, or PSOs for provider service organizations). Doctors are organizing into large multi-specialty group practices known as independent practice associations (IPAs) or group practices without walls. And insurers of all types are using innovative methods (some of which are thankfully still unabbreviated) for controlling medical expenditures.

The result of this cauldron of activity has been to make the health care lawyer's work much more demanding—and in demand. Each of these new organizations and innovative arrangements must be evaluated under a broad spectrum of private and public law. This chapter examines the bodies of law that are most relevant to these complex and novel transactions and organizational forms. In considers questions such as: When is an insurer or clinic engaged in the unlicensed corporate practice of medicine? Should physicians who receive capitation payments be regulated as de facto insurance companies? Should HMOs or joint ventures between doctors and hospitals be exempt from tax? What must nonprofit hospitals and insurers do in order to convert to for-profit status? Can hospitals reward physicians for generating income?

A.   THE CORPORATE PRACTICE OF MEDICINE

Perhaps the most threatening constraint on organizational innovation in health care is the corporate practice of medicine doctrine, which flatly declares that it is illegal for corporations to pay physicians for medical services. This peculiar doctrine can have devastating legal effects; it can result in the refusal to enforce contracts for medical services and it can lead to injunctions or even criminal sanctions against illegal business arrangements. It is also fundamental to the structure of the American health care delivery system in that it explains why physicians traditionally are financially independent from hospitals, each billing separately for their own services. This division reverberates throughout the system, reflected for instance, in the distinction between Blue Cross and Blue Shield and between Medicare Part A and Part B.

1. The Doctrine's Rationale

The rationale for the corporate practice doctrine is a confusing mixture of formalistic statutory reasoning and policy-based common law. The doctrine's statutory foundation rests on the medical practice act—the physician licensing statute in each state that makes it a criminal offense for anyone without a license to practice medicine. The doctrine reasons that when a corporation receives money from patients for a physician's medical services, the corporation is engaged in the practice of medicine. The doctrine then observes that corporations, not being natural persons, are ineligible for a medical license because they fail to meet the statutory prerequisites of sound moral character, a medical degree, and a passing score on the medical exam.

The corporate practice doctrine's common law foundation rests on the apprehension that physician employment will lead to debasement of the profession. Courts are concerned that employed physicians will focus unduly on earning a profit, that their patient loyalty will be subverted by their obligation to the corporation, and that their medical judgment will be countermanded by lay owners or administrators.

These rationales have been subjected to sustained criticism throughout its history. The statutory argument is formalistic sophistry in the view of many commentators. The argument is no more sound than the argument, say, that corporations who hire truck drivers are engaged in driving without a license. Clearly, if the *actions* of licensed physicians are to be attributed to the corporation, their licensed *status* should be as well.

The policy arguments, although more formidable, also are subject to critique. Physicians' financial dependence on corporations may present some marginally increased risk of profiteering and subverted patient loyalty but actual abuses of this nature are not well documented. The corporate practice doctrine arose at a time of widespread quackery in medicine practice, and the doctrine found its most convincing application in obviously shady cases, such as the corporate dentist who changed his name from Edgar to "Painless." Parker v. Board of Dental Examiners, 216 Cal. 285, 14 P.2d 67 (1932). Nevertheless, courts apply the doctrine even in the most upright circumstances and even when no lay owners or managers are involved. *See, e.g.,* Bartron v. Codington County, 2 N.W.2d 337 (S.D.1942) (illegal to operate a corporate clinic owned by physicians that provided services to indigent patients under contract with the county). As for policy concerns over controlling the course of treatment, admittedly it would be wrong for lay corporate managers to dictate the details of treatment, but such action would itself constitute a direct violation of the medical practice act regardless of who patients pay for medical services. Some degree of corporate influence is tolerable, however, and indeed is encouraged by liability law, which holds hospitals and HMOs responsible for the mistakes of their physicians. It seems contradictory to prohibit the very type of corporate influence that liability law seeks to encourage.

If there is a need for a separate corporate practice doctrine—other than simply to hold a corporation responsible for the acts of unlicensed practice actually committed by its *lay* employees—it is to prevent the possibility of physicians being influenced by corporate profit-making goals. This is viewed by many as naive idealism and out of step with modern public policy which sees a need for economic restraints on medical expenditures. Therefore, the remnants of this doctrine may stand in the path of innovative reform measures necessary to control health care spending. In the view of others, however, the doctrine's policy is far from anachronistic. Instead, the doctrine has renewed purpose in the modern environment when corporate and economic influences threaten to distort, if not overrun, medical judgment.

Regardless of one's views of the merits, courts have remained virtually steadfast in their recognition of the doctrine. Only two states have rejected it outright. Nevertheless, the extent of the doctrine's presence and enforcement varies widely from state to state. This is due in part to a number of exceptions that have been recognized on judicial and attorneys general opinions. It is also due to differing attitudes and practices among health care lawyers in different states.

2. The Doctrine's Survival

The absolutist nature of the corporate practice prohibition seems incredible given the many forms of corporate practice that pervade conventional medical establishments. Despite the doctrine's unqualified prohibition, physician employment is accepted and common practice in hospitals, government institutions, HMOs, and company clinics.

Explicit statutory exceptions exist for HMOs by virtue of their licensing statutes and the federal HMO Act (42 U.S.C. § 300e–10(a)). In addition, virtually every state has enacted a professional corporations law, which allows doctors, lawyers, and other professionals to enjoy the tax benefits of a corporate structure while operating in substance as a partnership. The modern versions of these laws cover limited liability corporations (LLCs) formed by licensed professionals.

Judicially-created exceptions exist in some, but not all, jurisdictions for non-profit institutions and for independent contracting in contrast with employment of physicians. Potentially the most important exception is for hospitals and other facilities that are licensed under a separate statutory scheme. Some courts, but not all, reason that this suffices to allow corporate payment of physicians within the scope of the facility's license. Berlin v.

Sarah Bush Lincoln Health Center, 688 N.E.2d 106 (Ill.1997).

Because most of the corporate practice case law dates from the 1930s, there has been some speculation in recent years that the doctrine may have died a quiet death during ensuing decades. However, corporate practice precedents survive in attorney general opinions and in established case law as "legal landmines, remnants of an old and nearly forgotten war, half-buried on a field fast being built up with new forms of health care organizations. Occasionally, usually at the instigation of those who resist the changes now taking place, one is detonated, with distressing results." Arnold Rosoff, *The Business of Medicine: Problems with the Corporate Practice Doctrine,* 17 Cumb.L.Rev. 485, 499 (1987). Instances of modern application include Morelli v. Ehsan, 737 P.2d 1030 (Wash.App.1987) (corporate practice doctrine bars enforcement of medical clinic partnership agreement by a lay partner/business manager); Conrad v. Medical Bd. of California, 55 Cal.Rptr.2d 901 (Cal.App.1996) (hospital district may not employ physicians).

B. INSURANCE AND HMO REGULATION

1. State Solvency Laws

In most states, insurance commissioners regulate the financial structure of insurance companies and the behavior of insurance sales forces, and in some states they also control the actual pricing and terms of insurance policies. Early on, litigation ensued over whether precursors to modern-day HMOs were subject to this regulatory authority. Courts initially held no, reasoning that HMOs bore less financial risk since they undertook the limited service obligation to deliver or arrange for care rather than the potentially unlimited financial obligation of indemnifying patients for the costs of whatever doctor or hospital they chose. Jordan v. Group Health Ass'n, 107 F.2d 239 (D.C.Cir.1939). Nevertheless, these and other laws, including the corporate practice prohibition, were seen as stumbling blocks to HMO development. For instance, many states had licensing statutes for Blue Cross that essentially required non-indemnity forms of insurance to have the support of the local medical society, and organized medicine has always opposed HMOs with all means at their disposal.

Most of the legal stumbling blocks were removed in a tide of legislation in the early 1970s embracing the HMO concept. The federal HMO Act 42 U.S.C. § 300e created grants and incentives for HMOs that voluntarily meet federal requirements, and preempted most of the obstructive state laws. States adopted HMO enabling statutes that regulate HMOs both as insurance companies and as health care delivery organizations. As a consequence, modern courts tend to find that HMO-type arrangements do constitute the business of insurance. See, e.g., State v. Abortion Information Agency, 330 N.Y.S.2d 927 (App.Div.1971), *aff'd* 334 N.Y.S.2d 174 (1972) (enjoining the operation of an abortion referral agency on the grounds that charging clients a single fee regardless of the expenses entailed constitutes the unauthorized business of insurance).

The overt regulation of HMOs creates a new regulatory dispute, namely, whether unlicensed HMO-type arrangements created by provider groups rather than insurance companies are subject to HMO regulation. Hospitals and physician groups are undertaking pre-paid capitation or other risk-bearing contracts with both HMOs (so-called "downstream capitation") and with employers ("direct contracting"). The first arrangement is designed to shift some or all of the insurance risk to the providers. The second is designed to cut out the insurer "middle-man" and to cater to self-insured employers. Under either arrangement, insurance regulators and licensed HMOs and insurers contend that providers are undertaking excessive financial risk for which they should have to meet solvency standards. Otherwise, these advocates for regulation claim there is an uneven competitive playing field which subjects licensed entities to greater costs and oversight. Provider groups respond that their risk is less than that of HMOs, for reasons similar to those advanced decades ago in *Jordan* supra.

So far, this dispute is unresolved. Federal regulators are adopting solvency standards for provider groups (called provider service organizations or PSOs) that accept Medicare patients on a capitated basis. These standards may or may not impose lower requirements on providers groups than on traditional insurers and HMOs. The response at the state level varies and is still evolving. Some states regulate only direct capitation contracts with employers and not sub-capitation contracts that are downstream from insurers or HMOs, reasoning that in the latter situation there is already regulatory protection for the ultimate consumer. However, ERISA preemption, discussed below, raises some doubt about whether capitation arrangements with self-funded employers are subject to state authority.

2.   The Federal HMO Act

Turning now to the federal regulatory arena, some commentators contend that the requirements for federal qualification imposed by the HMO Act of 1973 are so onerous that the Act has, paradoxically, done more to inhibit than to encourage HMO growth. They point to the fact that, despite the tremendous ability of HMOs to reduce unnecessary or marginally beneficial care, they have not substantially reduced the bottom line cost of insurance or imposed significant competitive discipline on the health insurance industry. Critics contend this is due in large part to the obstacles that the federal HMO Act placed in the path of using HMOs for rigorous cost containment.

There are two visions of how HMOs might improve health care. The *competitive vision* sees in HMOs the potential for translating their savings into lowered premiums, which will then force conventional insurance to search for innovative methods of cost containment. The *access vision* sees in HMOs the potential for translating their savings into increased services. The federal Act has followed the access model. It requires as a condition for federal qualification that HMOs engage in community rather than experience rating and that they provide comprehensive services with only nominal copayments from consumers. Thus, the main attraction for HMO enrollment has not been lower premiums for the employer but free check-ups, discounted prescriptions, and "first-dollar" coverage for the patient, all measures that tend to increase rather than restrain utilization. More importantly, the Act at first required employers to contribute equal amounts to HMO plans as to traditional indemnity plans, thereby removing any incentive the employer has to encourage HMO enrollment.

Congress addressed some of these defects in 1988 amendments to the Act. Federally-qualified HMOs are now allowed to provide up to 10 percent of their services through non-Plan physicians and to charge a "reasonable deductible" for these services. Also, the Act now liberalizes the definition of "community rating" to allow HMOs much greater flexibility in adjusting rates according to the health care experiences of different employee groups. The 1988 amendments replace the equal contribution requirement with one that allows employers reasonable variation in the amount they contribute to different plans and to different employee groups. The amendments also allow federally qualified HMOs to offer non-qualified product lines which contain leaner benefits.

As a consequence, HMOs are much more vigorously cost competitive in the 1990s than in earlier decades. Whereas before, they appeared to engage in "shadow pricing" by keeping their rates just below or in line with indemnity insurance, now they compete aggressively with each other and have imposed tough competitive discipline on the indemnity portion of the market. Some critics say that HMOs have achieved lower prices through "adverse selection" against indemnity insurance. There is some truth to the claim that older or sicker people tend to prefer indemnity insurance that preserves their choice of physician and maintains existing provider relationships. On the other hand, sicker patients might also prefer the more generous coverage, especially of drug benefits, found in HMOs.

3. Managed Care Patient Protections

The success of HMOs in containing costs leads to a renewed concern about their quality of care. While traditional fee-for-service reimbursement creates incentives for excessive *over*utilization, capitation can create incentives for excessive *under*utilization. HMOs also use gatekeeping and utilization review controls to restrict patients' choice of physicians and physicians' choice of treatment. Nevertheless, most broad based studies conclude that HMOs deliver care of equal or greater quality than under traditional fee-for-service insurance, and that HMO subscribers are generally well satisfied with the care they receive.

There are isolated instances of unscrupulous HMOs that have committed serious abuses, but most of these instances have occurred with HMOs participating in Medicaid and Medicare, which service patient populations that tend to be relatively captive in that they are less mobile, less able to complain, and less aware of their options to switch providers. These abuses are not as likely to occur if patients have an effective choice among insurers or are aware and able to exercise grievance and appeal rights.

These observations point to the ongoing debate over whether there should be more regulatory oversight of patient care in HMOs, or instead whether market forces and industry self-regulation are adequate safeguards. At the time of this writing, this debate is raging both in Congress and in the state legislatures, with numerous proposals under consideration. The flavor of the debate can be captured in the competing characterizations of "patient protections" or "bill of rights" versus "provider protections" or "anti-managed care backlash." Consider each of the following examples as either possible confirmation or refutation of these characterizations: (1) requiring a fair and speedy internal appeals process and notice of appeal rights; (2) requiring those who conduct utilization review to have a medical license in the state in which the treatment is rendered; (3) prohibiting so-called "drive-through deliveries" in which HMOs require mothers to leave the hospital within 24 hours of an uncomplicated child birth; (4) "any willing provider" laws that require HMOs to accept any physician who agrees to the plan's payment terms and meets its credentialing requirements; (5) requiring HMOs to engage in provider credentialing similar to that conducted by hospitals and giving physicians the right to challenge any adverse decisions; and (6) banning so-called "gag clauses" in managed care contracts with physicians, which prohibit physicians from making disparaging comments about the plan or from revealing trade secrets about payment terms or utilization review criteria.

C. ERISA PREEMPTION

The Employee Retirement Income Security Act of 1974 (ERISA), 29 U.S.C. 1144, is a federal statute that primarily regulates employer-sponsored pension plans to make sure that employers keep their promises and that funds are fairly administered. Incidentally, ERISA also covers other fringe benefits such as health insurance, but imposes very little regulation on them. In order to prevent inconsistent and overlapping state regulation, ERISA broadly preempts any state law that "relates to" an employer-sponsored fringe benefit plan.

We discuss ERISA preemption at this point because it incorporates the concept of the "business of insurance" discussed above and it limits the extent of state regulation of health insurance to a significant extent. However, it cannot be overly stressed that ERISA preemption permeates the landscape of health care law and public policy. As one health care scholar has noted, "Although in its text 'hospital' appears only once and 'physician' not at all, ERISA may be the most important law affecting health care in the United States." Wm. Sage, "Health Law 2000": The Legal System and the Changing Health Care Market, 15 Health Aff., No. 3, at 9 (Fall 1996).

ERISA preemption has major impact in three distinct places: (1) malpractice actions against HMOs; (2) contract claims for the denial of payment under health insurance; and (3) state regulation of how health insurance and HMO plans are sold and structured. The focus here is primarily on the third component, but this section also provides an overview that is useful for the other two topics. Moreover, it cannot be overemphasized that ERISA preemption is capable of cropping up almost anywhere in health law. For instance, each of the following are potentially preempted: physicians' contract actions against managed care plans that drop them from their networks; taxation of firms that assist self-insured employers in administering their health benefits; and state laws that limit health insurers' or employers' subrogation rights when employees' tort awards include medical expenses. See generally S. Law & B. Ensminger, Negotiating Physicians' Fees: Individual Patients or Society?, 61 N.Y.U. L. Rev. 1, 80–81 (1986) ("in this judicially constructed Alice in Wonderland world, any state seeking to regulate insurers' arrangements with physicians or providers must be prepared to litigate claims of ERISA preemption").

ERISA preemption is defined by the interaction of three distinct statutory phrases: (1) preemption applies to any state law that "relates to" employee benefits; (2) state authority is restored by an "insurance savings clause" that allows state regulation of the business of insurance; but (3) under the "deemer clause," states may not deem employers who self-fund rather than purchase insurance benefits to be engaged in the business of insurance. We will look at each of these phrases in turn.

The Supreme Court has stressed that the basic preemption provision, which reaches any state law that "relates to" an employee benefit plan, is to be construed very broadly. Prohibited state laws include both common law and statutory law. Thus, the Court has ruled that a state common law cause of action for bad faith and breach of contract in the denial of an insurance claim is pre-empted by ERISA. Pilot Life Ins. Co. v. Dedeaux, 107 S.Ct. 1549 (1987). However, a number of lower courts have ruled that garden variety malpractice suits against HMO physicians are not preempted, nor are vicarious liability theories against the HMO, since these implicate the employee benefit (health insurance) only indirectly. On the other hand, direct liability suits against HMOs claiming they made negligent coverage decisions or were negligent in selecting and supervising their physicians have been held to relate to employer-sponsored insurance and therefore are subject to preemption. One can also find decisions going the opposite way on both of these rulings. Moreover, one court suggested that this distinction between insurers' versus physicians' actions might be conflated if employers or insurers promise a certain level of quality from a managed care network. Then it could be argued that a physician's negligence constitutes a failure to deliver the promised employee benefit, much like a negligent insurance coverage decision. Dukes v. U.S. Healthcare, 57 F.3d 350 (3d Cir.1995). Whether this dictum will be accepted by other courts, and the full implications of the distinctions between vicarious and direct theories of HMO liability, are still very much in doubt.

The one notable decision that finds a health care law not potentially preempted is New York State Conference of Blue Cross & Blue Shield Plans v. Travelers Ins. Co., 514 U.S. 645 (1995). In *Travelers*, the Court held that ERISA does not preempt a New York statute that required hospitals to add a surcharge to their rates in order to fund a pool that reimbursed hospitals for the costs of treating patients without insurance. The plaintiffs in *Travelers* argued that the New York statute was preempted by ERISA because it made health insurance more expensive for employers to purchase, but the Supreme Court disagreed, holding that statutes that have "only an indirect economic effect on the relative costs of various health insurance packages." The Court emphasized, though, that it still supports a broad reading of "relates to."

The sweeping preemption provision is significantly limited by an "insurance savings clause" that reinstates state authority over matters that constitute the business of insurance. The Supreme Court has ruled that the same definition of insurance applies here as under the McCarran–Ferguson Act, which limits the application of other federal laws such as antitrust, securities, and banking regulation to insurance, so that these do not infringe on the traditional role of the states in regulating insurance. Thus, the definition of insurance becomes critical to determining the scope of state authority to regulate health care. For instance, in Metropolitan Life Insurance Co. v. Massachusetts, 471 U.S. 724 (1985), the Supreme Court held that a state law mandating the inclusion of mental health benefits in group health insurance falls within the savings clause and therefore is not preempted. In so holding, the Court established a three-part test, taken from McCarran–Ferguson Act precedents, for determining whether a given activity constitutes the business of insurance:

> First, whether the practice has the effect of transferring or spreading a policyholder's risk; second, whether the practice is an integral part of the policy relationship between the insurer and the insured; and third, whether the practice is limited to entities within the insurance industry.

471 U.S. at 743.

These three independent conditions severely limit the scope of the insurance savings clause and thus greatly expand the scope of ERISA's preemption provision. State law may regulate only those activities that fall directly within the core risk-spreading activity of insurance. This limitation excludes a broad array of important activity within the insurance industry. For example, the Supreme Court has held that an insurance company's determination of how much it is willing to pay a health care provider does not fall within the business of insurance because the decision does not relate directly to the policy holder. Group Life & Health Ins. Co. v. Royal Drug, 440 U.S. 205 (1979). Similarly, the Court has excluded from the business of insurance the process of verifying insurance claims because this occurs only after the policy has been issued. Union Labor Life Ins. Co. v. Pireno, 458 U.S. 119 (1982).

But wait, there's more! A third phrase in the statute declares that states may not deem a benefit plan itself to be insurance. As a result, another important policy effect of ERISA preemption is to promote employer self-insurance. The upshot of this "deemer clause" is that employers who self-fund medical benefits rather than purchase insurance for their employees are entirely exempt from state regulation, regardless of the scope of the savings clause. This provides a strong impetus for larger employers to self-insure their health care benefits, in order to reduce state regulation and avoid the cost of premium taxes. For instance, in *Metropolitan Life* supra, the Court observed that the state could not mandate that self-funded employers provide the same mental health benefits that are required of regulated insurers. Consequently, the number of employees covered by self-insured health care plans grew dramatically in the 1980s.

To recapitulate: (1) ERISA's preemption clause is extremely broad because so many state laws "relate to" employee benefits. (2) The insurance savings clause would reinstate most relevant state regulation, except for the fact that it has been given such a narrow construction. And, (3) regardless, for reasons just explained, self-insured health benefits may never be subjected to state regulation. The confusion surrounding this complicated scheme and the meaning of its various parts have deterred states from asserting more aggressive regulatory jurisdiction, even where that might be possible to do.

This would not be so troubling if it were not for the fact that substantive ERISA law imposes very little regulatory oversight to take the place of preempted state law. ERISA preemption makes perfect sense for private pension plans, which are closely monitored by the substantive provisions in ERISA, but other employee benefits were added to ERISA as a legislative after-thought, and so ERISA is not designed to regulate or enforce them. For these benefits, ERISA creates a severe regulatory vacuum by failing to fill the void it creates. To illustrate, in McGann v. H & H Music Co., 946 F.2d 401 (5th Cir. 1991), the court held that it could do nothing about a self-funded employer that virtually eliminated its insurance coverage of treatment for AIDS shortly after it discovered an employee was afflicted. The court observed that ERISA was not intended to guarantee any particular level of benefits but only to enforce the benefits promised, and here the employer had not promised never to change its insurance benefits. Another example of limited state authority comes from the few states that have attempted to deal with the problem of uninsured workers by mandating that all employers offer health benefits. These laws have been held to violate ERISA preemption.

Those who oppose mandated benefits and mandated employer coverage as unwarranted incursions in the health insurance market view these restrictions on state authority as good public policy. Others obviously disagree. The arena in which this debate is presently the most contentious is with respect to malpractice actions against HMOs. Where these are preempted, ERISA provides very limited remedy. Because it was designed to enforce the contractual promise of monetary pension benefits, ERISA allows only injunctive and direct contract damages (that is, the value of the promised benefits), but no remedies for personal injury or pain and suffering that are the consequence of a breach of promised benefits. Mertens v. Hewitt Associates, 508 U.S. 248 (1993). This makes sense for pension plans, but not for the breach of health insurance, which results in the denial of medical care. Therefore, various legislative proposals have been made in Congress to create a federal HMO liability law.

Another indication that the ERISA vacuum is starting to leak is found in the Health Insurance Portability and Accountability Act of 1996, which for the first time requires even self-funded insurers to offer a few specified benefits (limited mental

health coverage, and at least 48 hours of hospitalization for uncomplicated child-birth). Some commentators see this as a harbinger of eventual federal take-over of health insurance regulation. Only
time will tell.

D. CHARITABLE TAX EXEMPTION

Most hospitals are organized as nonprofit corporations. Standing alone, nonprofit status confers no
special tax advantage; it means merely that no
capital stock is issued and no dividends are paid.
However, many nonprofit corporations, including
hospitals, are eligible for various forms of both
federal and state tax relief because they also qualify
for classification as charitable organizations. Principally, section 501(c)(3) of the federal tax code provides that "corporations . . . organized and operated
exclusively for religious, charitable, scientific . . . or
educational purposes, . . . no part of the earnings of
which inures to the benefit of any private . . .
individual," shall be exempt from income tax. Nonprofit hospitals are also uniformly exempt from
local property taxes and state income taxes. Because
nonprofit institutions historically have dominated
the health care sector, the requirements for maintaining tax exemption have a profound effect on the
organization and operation of health care facilities.
The following discussion explores three aspects of
tax exemption: the basic eligibility for charitable
status, the prohibition against private inurement,
and the effect of receiving income that is unrelated
to the institution's charitable purpose. At the end,

this section also considers the conversion of no-profit facilities to for-profit status.

1. The Basis for Tax Exemption

a. *Hospital Services*

Resolving the basic question of why hospitals are considered charitable organizations is more difficult than might first be expected. Hospitals originated during the 18th and 19th centuries as almshouses for the poor, essentially warehousing the impoverished sick who, prior to modern medicine, were not fortunate enough to afford treatment at home. These desperate institutions were usually operated under the auspices of a religious order and were supported almost entirely by charitable donations of time, money and property.

Consistent with these historical origins, the IRS initially required charitable hospitals to provide free care "to the extent of their financial ability." Rev. Rul. 56–185. However, as insurance became widespread for the middle class in the post-World War II era and as the social welfare programs of the 1960s extended broad financial support to the elderly and poor, the optimistic attitude arose that there would soon be no demand for charity care and no need for charitable donations.

How, then, were hospitals to justify continued charitable status? The IRS responded in 1969 by modifying its position to allow hospitals to receive tax-exempt status merely on the conditions that they not discriminate among paying patients and they treat all indigent *emergency* patients for free. Rev.Rul. 69–545. More recently, in 1983, the IRS went a step further and ruled that even free emergency care is not required if an emergency room is not needed or appropriate at a hospital (for example, because it is a highly specialized facility such as an eye and ear hospital). Rev.Rul. 83–187.

Under these rulings hospitals no longer have to provide any specific amount of health care free of charge to the poor in order to qualify under § 501(c)(3) of the Internal Revenue Code. This result is not entirely unprecedented. To be considered "charitable" under the tax code an organization need not necessarily be a charity in the everyday sense of assisting the poor. Many educational and scientific organizations exempt from tax and supported by tax deductible contributions provide no or few services to the poor; serving the poor has never been the only activity accepted as "charitable" under either the tax code or the traditional law of charitable trusts. The IRS consulted precedents from the law of charitable trusts to determine that advancing health provides a separate and sufficient basis for favorable tax treatment, apart from charity care. In essence, hospital care is treated like education—as being a *per se* charitable service.

This shift in policy was opposed by welfare advocacy groups who feared that the naive optimism of the 1960s, which thought the demand for charity care would be fully met by Medicare and Medicaid, was wrong. However, legal challenges to the IRS failed in 1976 when the Supreme Court ruled that patients do not have standing to challenge a hospital's tax status. Simon v. Eastern Ky. Welfare Rights Org., 426 U.S. 26 (1976). As a result, many hospitals faced with other pressing financial problems have begun to abandon or diminish their traditional commitment to treating the poor.

A similar battle has occurred at the state level, where advocacy groups have found allies in local taxing authorities hoping to secure new sources of property tax revenue. While state courts have usually followed the federal lead, one notable case took a sharply different tack. In Utah County v. Intermountain Health Care, Inc., 709 P.2d 265 (Utah 1985), the court revoked the property tax exemption of two nonprofit hospitals because they failed both to provide sufficient services to the poor and to attract a significant level of donations. The court found that less than one percent of the hospitals' services were provided free as charity care, and that one of the hospitals had "dumped" indigent patients from its emergency room. No other court has gone this far; however a few states, notably Texas and Pennsylvania, passed legislation that requires nonprofit hospitals to make a significant "gift to the community" in some form of free services.

b. Other Health Care Institutions

Hospitals are not the only health care institutions concerned with tax exempt status. Nonprofit health maintenance organizations (HMOs), outpatient clinics, and pharmacies have also sought to maintain exempt status. When confronted with these nonhospital health care services, federal and state tax policy tends to take a distinctly less welcoming attitude.

Despite the IRS acceptance of health care as a *per se* charitable enterprise, it has been reluctant to confer tax exempt status on nonprofit physician groups, HMOs, or other medical enterprises. For instance, the tax court has ruled that a nonprofit pharmacy organized to sell discount prescription drugs to the elderly does not pursue a charitable purpose. Such an enterprise clearly serves the community's health care needs; nevertheless, the tax court ruled that an exemption was not warranted because the sale of drugs at cost is a "substantial commercial activity ... in competition with profit-making drugstores." Federation Pharmacy Services, Inc., 72 T.C. 687 (1979). This commerciality standard obviously cannot be reconciled with the *per se* theory that is applied to hospitals, since they too are in direct competition with for-profit firms.

The IRS has also grappled with whether nonprofit health insurers and HMOs qualify for exemption. In 1986, Congress withdrew exemption from Blue Cross/Blue Shield because it viewed the sale of insurance as an inherently commercial activity. I.R.C. § 501(m). How should HMOs then be treated? At first, the IRS took the position that HMOs are merely another form of insurance and therefore not entitled to exemption. However, under pressure from contrary tax court rulings, the IRS adopted a position that seeks to classify which HMOs are more like hospitals, and which are more like insurers. Roughly speaking, the current IRS position is that staff model HMOs are more like hospitals because they directly deliver health care services, and so they can qualify for exemption if they are sufficiently open to the public at large and provide some measure of free services, especially if they own and operate nonprofit hospitals with open emergency rooms. However, IPA or network model HMOs are not exempt, even if they meet these same standards, because they merely "arrange for" health care services. In the leading case of Geisinger Health Plan v. Commissioner, 985 F.2d 1210 (3d Cir.1993), the Third Circuit sustained this position.

A related issue of dispute has been whether integrated delivery systems (IDSs) can receive charitable exemption. They are composed of large networks of physicians and hospitals and they sell insurance, so they might fit within any of several different precedents. For the most part, the IRS has been accommodating to IDSs, applying to them essentially the same tests as apply to hospitals, especially if the network is built around a large nonprofit hospital that also supports education and research functions. However, in one respect, the IRS rulings have made exemption difficult for integrated systems. The IRS initially ruled that exempt status would be questioned if more than 20 percent of the governing board is composed of physicians who practice in the system. This ruling was based on obscure precedents from tax exempt bond financing, and is premised on the idea that physicians have a conflict of interest that might potentially cause them to manage the system for their own professional benefit rather than for the community's benefit. The consequence, however, is that many integrated systems opted against nonprofit status because they felt they could not operate and recruit effectively unless physicians were given a significant leadership role. Under harsh criticism, the IRS relented on the 20 percent guideline and now allows up to 49 percent physician membership on the board, as long as physicians' salary decisions are made by an independent committee and there are other conflict-of-interest protections in place.

The sharp dichotomy between exemption for hospitals and exemption for other health care services reflects the reality that neither state nor federal taxing authorities actually accept the proposition that health care is a per se charitable purpose, just as they would be unlikely to exempt a nonprofit bookstore despite the per se exemption for "education" that is explicit in the statute. Instead, these authorities are searching for an alternative exemption rationale to differentiate between those health care services that deserve a tax subsidy and those that do not. Although the basis of individual rulings may (or may not) be fairly clear, the overarching theory of charitable exemption remains elusive.

2. Inurement to Private Benefit

In addition to serving a charitable purpose, health care institutions must comply with several operational requirements to be eligible for tax exemption. The principal threat to exempt status is the private inurement prohibition: "*no* part of the [hospital's] net earnings [may] inure[ ] to the private benefit of *any* private shareholder or individual." Code § 501(c) (emphasis added). For example, in the leading federal decision, the court found that restricting hospital access exclusively to a small group of physicians undermines exempt status because it converts the hospital into essentially a private workshop rather than a public facility. Harding Hospital, Inc. v. United States, 505 F.2d 1068 (6th Cir.1974). The court also cited as evidence of private inurement: (1) the hospital's provision of office space, medical equipment, and clerical services to staff physicians at below-market rates; and (2) the hospital's payment of a large management fee to the doctors for hospital supervision.

The IRS has identified several other activities that may jeopardize exempt status. Hospitals frequently offer a package of benefits to new physicians in order to attract them to understaffed rural areas, benefits such as discounted office space and a guaranteed minimum income. The IRS has indicated that such inducements may or may not constitute private inurement, depending on the reasonableness and necessity of the amounts offered in individual cases. Similarly, the IRS has stated that it may be legitimate for a hospital to act as a general partner with physicians in a venture to construct a medical facility, even though by so doing the hospital contributes substantial capital and places its assets at risk, but such joint venture activity requires a highly individualized determination of the value of the *quid pro quo* in each case.

Where the IRS has drawn the line is at joint ventures designed solely to give physicians a financial stake in the success of an existing department or facility. This can occur through arrangements that blatantly sell to physicians for a nominal amount a portion of the revenue stream produced by their hospitalized patients. In General Counsel Memorandum 39862 (Dec. 2, 1991), the IRS ruled that this constitutes obvious private inurement because there is no shared investment risk in a new facility or service, only a thinly disguised attempt to encourage physicians to make greater use of one hospital rather than another. This is a motive the IRS does not consider to be a benefit to the community, even though it clearly does benefit the hospital.

3. Unrelated Business Income

A matter of less serious concern, but still of substantial importance to tax-exempt organizations, is the treatment of income from activities unrelated to the entity's exempt purpose. Such unrelated business income does not jeopardize the organizations' *overall* exempt status unless it rises to a substantial level in comparison with overall operations. Nevertheless, unrelated business income is subject to separate taxation. For instance, income from a hospital gift shop would never be large enough to threaten taxation of the hospital's entire income, but if gift shop income were considered "unrelated" to a hospital's exempt purpose, the gift shop income itself would be taxed. The sources of such potentially unrelated income in hospitals are numerous and significant enough to have generated a number of rulings.

The Code provision on unrelated business income, section 513(a), defines such income as that "which is not substantially related [to the] ... purpose or function constituting the basis for exemption, ... except that such term does not include any trade or business which is carried on ... by the organization primarily for the convenience of its ... patients or employees." Consider how this definition might apply to income from hospital gift shops, cafeteria sales, and parking lot receipts—services that are patronized largely by visitors. The IRS has found these sources of income to be exempt. This result is easily justified under the "convenience for patients and employees" exception, but the Service has chosen to rest this result in the strained reasoning that such sales are substantially related to patient care by virtue of the therapeutic benefits of patient visitation. The IRS takes the opposite stance when it addresses income from hospital pharmacies and laboratories derived from nonhospital patients. The Service has ruled that this income is *un*related to a hospital's exempt purpose, even though it is patient care income from patients of doctors on the medical staff whose offices are maintained next door in a tax-exempt office complex.

4. Hospital Reorganization, Diversification, and Conversion of Status

a. *Reorganization and Diversification*

The tumultuous environment that prevails in the health care industry is prompting widespread experimentation with organizational innovations. Virtually every hospital of any significant size has undergone some type of corporate reorganization in recent years. Typically, a nonprofit hospital will segregate its various functions, some for-profit and some nonprofit, and incorporate them into separate entities, all under the common ownership of a holding company. Such corporate restructuring raises many of the tax issues discussed so far, such as whether a particular hospital function (say, laundry) standing alone will support an exemption and, if not, whether it is sufficiently related to an exempt function to be free from the unrelated business income tax if organized as part of the hospital corporate entity.

The tax consequences of hospital diversification are especially important in the modern business climate. The rampant excess hospital capacity and shrinking patient service revenues have caused hospitals to venture into all sorts of new enterprises. Some are directly related to health care, such as nursing homes and home health services. Others are far afield, such as athletic clubs, real estate development, and day care centers. Sophisticated hospital counsel, in deciding how to structure these ventures, must not only consider the tax problems surveyed here but also the potentially countervailing effects of government reimbursement regulations and certificate of need requirements. Tax law might prompt a hospital to internalize a new venture in order to claim it as related business income, but doing so might necessitate a certificate of need or might adversely affect reimbursement under Medicare, Medicaid, or state rate regulatory programs (topics addressed elsewhere in this book).

b. Conversion to For–Profit Status

Another type of restructuring that has swept the industry is conversion to for-profit status. Despite the benefits of tax exemption, many hospitals, HMOs, and Blue Cross plans are finding it more attractive to forgo nonprofit status. Perhaps this is prompted by the demands of maintaining charitable tax exemption, or perhaps it is that for-profit status allows better access to capital markets by permitting equity investment. Another possibility is that members of nonprofit hospital and Blue Cross boards, who often view their volunteer positions as community service, are finding the modern climate too difficult to continue operations with a truly charitable mission. For whatever reason, nonprofit conversions are becoming legion, and they can generate enormous public controversy. The same is true for public hospitals, which are increasingly converting to private status, often to avoid restrictive enabling legislation that keeps them from entering into the contractual arrangements that are necessary to compete in a managed care environment.

Conversion of status can occur through several different forms. The simplest is for the nonprofit corporation or municipal government to sell its principal asset to a for-profit entity so that now it owns cash rather than a hospital or insurance company. Somewhat more complex is to retain ownership of the facility but enter into a long-term management contract with a for-profit firm to run the hospital, rewarding it based on a percentage of the profits. Either type of transaction raises a host of corporate or municipal law issues that must be resolved.

The first issue is whether the transaction is within the corporate powers or instead is *ultra vires*. This issue arises because the articles of incorporation for nonprofit entities, and the authorizing legislation for government entities, frequently limit the purposes for which the entity can operate. For instance, if these governing documents authorize hospital operations but not health care or charitable purposes more generally, then the entity has difficulty justifying selling a hospital and devoting the proceeds to some other use. Similarly, if donors to the hospital have restricted their gifts to particular uses, such as supporting a particular facility, then any conversion of the assets would violate a promise made to donors who may be long-since deceased.

One way nonprofits can avoid the restrictions of the *ultra vires* doctrine is to invoke the concept of *cy pres* from the law of charitable trusts. The *cy pres* doctrine addresses situations where it is no longer possible or feasible to carry out the original terms of a charitable gift, and so courts can authorize a change in the purpose to the next closest use. Whether the intensely competitive climate of modern health care is a compelling enough change in circumstances to force a charitable hospital to abandon its nonprofit status is a question on which few courts have ruled, but modern trust law decisions generally apply the *cy pres* doctrine somewhat more liberally than in the past. However authorized, once charitable assets are sold, then these same rules control how the proceeds can be used. Most nonprofit hospitals, HMOs, and Blue Cross plans have chosen to use the proceeds to fund a charitable foundation to advance community health.

The next issue, then, is whether the amounts received in the transaction are sufficient. This refers to the fiduciary duties of care and loyalty that all corporate managers, including nonprofit board members, owe in their corporate governance. The risk that exists in nonprofit settings is that the absence of any oversight from owners and shareholders with a stake in the transaction may make board members lax in their negotiations. Even more troubling, the acquiring for-profit firm may undermine nonprofit board members' loyalty by holding out the prospect of rich personal rewards if the transaction goes forward. For instance, board members have been offered lucrative positions or bargain basement ownership shares in the new for-profit entity, which obviously encourages them to approve the transaction. Fiduciary law that applies to nonprofit and for-profit corporations alike prohibits such conflicts of interest and can be used to void tainted transactions.

Resolving these issues requires that nonprofit assets be fairly valued in conversion transactions. Fair valuation of nonprofit assets is a difficult analytical exercise, however, on which opinions differ widely. One possibility is a "hard asset, depreciated value" approach, which looks at what it would cost to build or replace the assets. This tends to produce a fairly low valuation because it ignores the firm's good will and established reputation in the market. A second approach is to value the enterprise as an ongoing business, but even this produces a valuation that is often much lower than the speculative value that can result from the sale of its stock. There are numerous instances of hospitals and insurers whose stock market value a year or two after their conversion ends up being many times higher than the sales price. This creates a strong impression that the original price was greatly depressed due to a lack of arms length or conflict-free negotiations. On the other hand, a good bit of this value can be attributed to the mere fact of the conversion. The enterprise is simply worth more now that it can have equity investors and its management is in different hands. It is not clear who should get credit for this added value that is created by the transaction itself.

The number and difficulty of issues presented by a conversion transaction raises the further question of who is in a position to make sure they are properly resolved. Owing to the lack of shareholder oversight, state law usually gives the attorney general authority to challenge in court any nonprofit transaction that appears questionable. In the past, careful counsel sometimes requested and paid for an attorney general to bring a nominal challenge simply in order to gain the court's approval so the transaction cannot later be invalidated. More recently, however, attorneys general have posed real opposition to conversions, reflecting the public's hostility to losing the nonprofit character of valued community institutions. In a number of states, legislatures have required approval by attorneys general or administrative agencies before conversions can proceed, and attorneys general themselves have been proactive in promulgating guidelines and negotiating the terms under which they will approve, or not oppose, conversions.

E.   REFERRAL FEE PROHIBITIONS

1.   Sources of Law

Paying health care providers purely as an inducement to refer patients has long been considered unethical and inappropriate. Kickbacks for ordering or recommending treatment have been shown in various empirical studies to distort judgment about whether services are necessary and who are the better providers. These costs are borne not only by the patients affected, but also by the public and private insurance that pays for the care. Accordingly, referral fees are prohibited by several sources of law.

Fee splitting is frequently listed in medical practice acts as one basis for professional discipline. The payment of referral fees also constitutes a felony under some state statutes. *E.g.,* Cal.Bus. & Prof. Code § 650. But the federal law contains the most prominent prohibition. The anti-fraud and abuse provisions of the Medicare and Medicaid programs, paraphrased, declare: anyone who receives or pays any remuneration directly or indirectly, overtly or covertly, in cash or in kind for the referral of a patient to a person for the furnishing of any item or service for which payment may be made under Medicare or Medicaid is guilty of a felony punishable by five years imprisonment or $25,000, or both. 42 U.S.C. § 1320a–7b(b). Referral fees are also prohibited by a federal statute known as the "Stark law," named for Rep. Fortney "Pete" Stark who championed it. The Stark law prohibits Medicare and Medicaid from paying for any services that physicians render or order through entities that they have a financial relationship with. 42 U.S.C. § 1395nn. This is meant to prohibit so-called "self-referral fees," that is, incentives for physicians to send patients to entities they own or receive money from.

So, the message is clear: referral fees are bad. Unfortunately, confusion reigns over precisely what this means. Implicit or explicit referral incentives pervade most accepted and legitimate relationships in medicine, so it is far from clear which are prohibited and which are not. For instance, it could be argued that simply offering a discount in the sale of medical services constitutes a sort of self-referral fee since the discount might, quite literally, be characterized as a "kickback" from the seller to the purchaser intended to induce the purchaser to select that seller. As another example of completely innocent referral incentives, a hospital's granting of medical staff privileges might be viewed as a form of consideration meant to encourage physicians to admit patients to the hospital. Yet it would be ludicrous to contend that this cornerstone of the health care delivery system is fundamentally unethical and criminally illegal. It is necessary, then, to search for some analytical guide to distinguish illicit referral incentives from acceptable practices.

2. Earned Versus Unearned Fees

The analytical distinction that provides the greatest assistance in determining which referral incentives are illegal is to distinguish between earned and unearned fees. Earned fees are those in exchange for a legitimate, non-referral service of fair market value. Unearned fees are any that do not have a non-referral quid pro quo or that are in excess of the fair market value for the exchange service.

This is a quite sensible and workable approach that avoids messy inquiries into subjective motives. For example, radiologists and pharmacists can be required to pay hospitals a reasonable percentage of the revenues they generate from hospital patients in exchange for the hospital providing equipment and staffing, despite the fact that this results in the physicians paying the hospital in proportion to the amount of business received from hospital patients. Blank v. Palo Alto–Stanford Hospital Center, 44 Cal.Rptr. 572 (Cal.App.1965), held that a radiologist's payment to the hospital of two-thirds of his receipts does not constitute fee splitting because "the evidence sustains the conclusion that the portion of the fees received was commensurate with the expenses ... incurred by the hospital in connection with furnishing the diagnostic facilities.... Under these circumstances there is no illegality."[1] In other words, the splitting of radiology fees was valid despite its direct and immediate relationship to the level of referrals from the hospital because, so long as the fees were in fair exchange for legitimate services, they were not "as compensation for referring patients."

Unfortunately, referral fee interpretations frequently stray from this analytical path. The decision that has caused the most concern under federal law is United States v. Greber, 760 F.2d 68 (3d Cir.1985). It addressed a clinical laboratory's prac-

1. Note that the outcome may be different for a pharmacy, because with the rental of space rather than equipment, the cost to the hospital does not vary in proportion to the amount of business. Therefore, in contrast with radiology, the California Attorney General has viewed with suspicion a percentage-of-receipts lease for a hospital pharmacy. 53 Cal.Atty.Gen.Op. 117, 119 (1970).

tice of paying "interpretation fees" to compensate physicians for evaluating their patients' test results, a well-recognized disguise for a kickback. The court sustained a criminal conviction, observing that the fee paid exceeded the value of the interpretation services and that some doctors were paid even though they didn't perform any service. Although this decision was clearly correct on its facts, the court made a broad and troubling pronouncement that reached far beyond the particulars of the case: "if the payments were intended to induce the physician to use [the laboratory's] services, the statute was violated, *even if the payments were also intended to compensate for professional services.*" 760 F.2d at 72 (emphasis added). *Greber* thus leaves in doubt what analytical guide should be used to reach a sensible interpretation of this broad and ambiguous concept.

Additional guidance comes from several different sources. Under the Medicare/Medicaid anti-kickback statute, DHHS is instructed to promulgate safe-harbor regulations "specifying payment practices that shall not be treated as a criminal offense under [the referral fee statute]." These safe-harbor regulations rely heavily on the fair market value concept. For instance, they allow physicians to invest in medical enterprises if they do so on terms that are offered to non-physician investors, and they allow hospitals to rent space to physicians on terms that are "consistent with fair market value in arms-length transactions." Similar guidance is contained in the Stark statute itself, through a number of complex statutory definitions and exceptions that capture the same concepts. However, these regulations and statutory provisions are narrowly drawn to cover only a limited number of discrete transactions, and only those that are generally accepted to be beyond approach. They do not offer more general analytical guidance for resolving innovative arrangements that are not yet in common use or those that are in use but that are more difficult to judge. This has led to continuing criticism that these laws stifle productive innovation or cause legitimate and well-meaning ventures to operate under a cloud of potential illegality.

Responding to this criticism, Congress has recently taken two important steps. First, it has required the enforcement agencies to create more sweeping exemptions for incentive arrangements within managed care or capitated payment systems. This recognizes the fact that productivity or inflationary incentives may be an important safeguard to counteract larger cost containment pressures. Second, Congress has required the enforcement agencies to institute a process for obtaining transaction-specific advisory rulings, much like is done under tax and antitrust laws. Although this process is still new, the initial rulings indicate that the enforcement agencies will continue to take a very cautious view of which arrangements are permissible. For instance, in one of the early rulings, a hospital was told that it could not restock supplies on independent ambulances that served its emergency room, for fear that overly generous restocking could be used to encourage ambulance drivers to select one hospital over another.

F.   SUMMARY

The array of transactions and organizational structures among doctors, hospitals and insurers is subject to a complex tapestry of legal doctrines. The health care lawyer's job is made more difficult because these multiple bodies of law often give sharply inconsistent signals about which particular arrangements are legally preferred. No one arrangement is ideal, either from a legal or a business planning perspective. To gain some sense of the overall picture that results, consider the following chart, which displays a rough guide for how various business and legal perspectives would regard three different methods a hospital might pursue for closer affiliation with physicians. Suppose the affiliation were undertaken either to market a comprehensive managed care insurance plan, or, less ambitiously, to establish an outpatient clinic. This chart indicates whether each business or legal factor would view each arrangement favorably (+), negatively (-), or in a neutral/mixed (/) fashion.

This rough outline is only a general approximation and is subject to some dispute, but for what it is worth, here is what these labels are based on:

	Physician Autonomy	Clinical and Financial Integration	Corporate Practice of Medicine	Antitrust	Referral Fee Law	Tax Exempt
Foundation Plan (The hospital's corporate parent buys out physician practices and employs the physicians)	-	+	-	+	+	+
Physician-Hospital Organization (PHO) (Hospital and several physician groups form joint-venture partnership, contribute equal capital, and split the proceeds)	-	-	-	-	-	-
Management Services Organization (MSO) (Hospital contracts with independent physicians to provide office management services and to act as negotiating agent with insurers/employers)	+	-	+	-	-	-

- Physician autonomy favors looser forms of integration whereas management concerns favor tighter integration, and so these two dimensions run in opposite directions.

- The *corporate practice doctrine* favors MSOs because payments aren't for medical services. The corporate practice doctrine is most clearly violated by the Foundation model, so that can be used only if state law creates an exception for nonprofits or for hospitals. PHOs may be safe if physicians and hospitals bill and collect separately.

- *Antitrust* favors the Foundation model because it is a single entity, whereas the MSO is the least integrated and therefore potentially closest to price fixing. The PHO would depend on how the particular arrangement falls under the DOJ/FTC guidelines. These considerations don't take account of market share (merger) or boycott (exclusion) issues.

- *Referral fee laws* also favor the Foundation model because payments occur within an integrated entity where it is less obvious that any "referral" occurs, and for which various exceptions exist. PHOs do the worst under the Stark law, although not too badly under the anti-kickback statute as long as the investment arrangement is properly structured. MSOs run the risk of both under-and over-compensating for services, thereby creating potential referral incentives in either direction.

● *Tax exemption* favors hospitals and disfavors doctors. MSOs don't provide medical services and
  therefore have only a tenuous connection with
  the health care exemption.

*

PART III

ETHICAL ISSUES IN PATIENT CARE DECISIONS

In Part III we shift our focus to issues that arise in individual patient care decisions. This Part addresses certain recurring ethical dilemmas that confront physicians and hospital administrators. We begin in Chapter 6 by looking at the problem of defining death, which is related to how organs are harvested and distributed for transplantation since the dead are a critical source of organ donations. A clear grasp of the definition of death is also important to understanding issues that arise in the termination of life-sustaining treatment, which is the subject of Chapter 7. Chapter 8 then shifts our attention to the beginning of life, examining the ethical dilemmas arising in two selected areas of reproductive medicine: advanced reproductive technologies, and maternal-fetal conflict. While Part III provides a comprehensive overview of the relevant law, it often goes beyond the law to survey the philosophical and policy debates that permeate these questions.

CHAPTER 6

DEFINING DEATH AND TRANSPLANTING ORGANS

A. DEFINING DEATH

Death is not necessarily a univocal concept. Medically, death is a diagnosis. Philosophically, death is a moral concept. People's interests, and the obligations owed them, are usually thought to depend upon certain qualities possessed only by the living. In religious traditions, death may simply be a transition, a time when the soul leaves the body for another world.

Legally, many different things may turn upon a determination of death: whether a homicide has been committed; when organs can be harvested for transplantation; when burial, cremation, or autopsy can occur; the sequence in which wills should be probated; when a spouse can remarry; whether a party has standing to bring an action in his own right. In theory one might look to varying criteria for the definition of death, depending on the legal purpose for which the inquiry is made, for example, to determine whether to remove a heart versus whether a homicide has been committed. The law, however, has ordinarily accepted the medical diagnosis as dispositive for all purposes. In the 1970s, a change in the medical view of death was widely and rather quickly adopted by the law. This has prompted an ongoing debate over the proper standard and its implications.

1. Cardiopulmonary Criteria

The traditional criterion of death was the cessation of respiration and circulation. The shortcomings of this "cardiopulmonary" definition emerged with the advent of technology capable of artificially sustaining one's "vital signs" for days, weeks, or even longer, even though the brain has ceased functioning. Since such persons breathe and circulate blood, the cardiopulmonary standard precluded their being considered "dead" despite their general lack of responsiveness to any stimuli and their inability to sustain even a *vegetative* existence without the technology. In a precursor to the current "futility" debate (see ch. 7.E), physicians and ethicists questioned the legal standard that treated patients as "alive" simply because some cells or organs continued to live, when their bodies had permanently ceased all capacity to function as integrated wholes. Of at least equal importance, treating such people as alive prevented effective retrieval of their organs for transplantation. While the need to procure organs, by itself, is not sufficient justification for altering the medical definition of death, it provided an important motivation for rethinking it.

2. Neurological Criteria: Whole Brain Death

The solution to these difficulties has been to redefine death so that it is properly diagnosed when there has been either a permanent cessation of all respiratory and circulatory function *or* when the brain has died. The modern legal rule, applied in most states, is stated in the Uniform Determination of Death Act, as proposed in 1981 by the President's Commission for the Study of Ethical Problems in Medicine and Biomedical and Behavioral Research:

> An individual who has sustained either (1) irreversible cessation of circulatory and respiratory function, or (2) irreversible cessation of all functions of the entire brain, including the brain stem, is dead. A determination of death must be made in accordance with accepted medical standards.

All states, by statute or judicial decision, have accepted some form of the whole-brain death criterion.

Note that the rule requires *whole* brain death, "including the brain stem." Anatomically, the brainstem is an extension of the spinal cord into the base of the skull; functionally, it is responsible for most of the vegetative functions essential to maintaining life, such as respiration, swallowing, and sleep-awake cycles (in contrast with the upper brain, which controls consciousness, thought, feeling, and memory). Thus death of the brainstem means loss of the ability to maintain respiration spontaneously. Without respiration, the heart (which is *not* directly dependent on the brain to continue beating) will die from a lack of oxygen, and circulation will stop. Brain death, therefore, inevitably leads to the termination of cardiopulmonary functions, unless respiration is artificially maintained.

Because in the normal course of events the three systems (heart, lung and brain) fail more or less simultaneously, regardless of which one fails first, the two formulations are sometimes characterized not as different *concepts* of death, but as alternative *criteria* for measuring the same underlying status—the permanent "disintegration" of the organism as a whole, reflected in the cessation of integrated functioning among these three essential, interdependent systems. Some argue, however, that brain death *is* conceptually different, in a manner that is not simply an alternative to cardiopulmonary death. Due to the brain's unique primacy in integrating the functions of the organism as a whole, its death is the "real" (or at least, the most important) criterion for the demise of a person. Without a living brain, some tissue may be alive, but the *person* is not. In this view respiration and circulation retain validity only as a concession to lay perceptions of human vitality, or to diagnostic simplicity .

Whatever the conceptual model, acceptance of brain death is quite important as a practical matter, for it enables the transplantation of organs essential to life. Under current law, taking essential organs from someone who is still alive, even with his consent, is homicide, but we cannot wait for the donor's heart to stop before taking it, since it will then not beat for the recipient either. The donor's other organs will also soon die from the lack of circulation. An acceptable donor of a heart, liver, or both kidneys must be dead, but still breathing and circulating blood.[1] The legal acceptance of whole brain death permits this.

Conceivably, one could achieve the same result in other ways, for instance by making an exception to the "dead donor" rule for terminally ill patients, or by modifying the cardiopulmonary criterion to refer to loss of *spontaneous* respiratory function, but there are problems with each of these approaches. Modifying the dead donor rule would breach the fundamental prohibition of suicide and would pose difficulties in defining terminal status. Modifying the cardiopulmonary standard would pose similar difficulties in determining whether the inability to breathe on one's own is "irreversible;" some people can be "weaned" from ventilators, but it is difficult and harrowing to determine who they are by trial and error. Adopting a brain death standard accomplishes the same result with much greater diagnostic certainty, since a person who has no brain-stem activity also has no spontaneous respiration. Moreover, brain death is morally appealing to those who believe it is conceptually superior to adopt a criterion that focuses on the centrality of the brain in the integration of the organism.

1. This may be less true now than in the 1970s, since new medical techniques (e.g., infusing cold fluids into a cadaver) help to keep organs viable even after cardiopulmonary death. Also, it is possible to terminate life support in an operating room where organs can be removed moments after cardiopulmonary functions cease.

3. Neurological Criteria: Upper Brain Death

Laypersons sometimes think that brain death occurs simply with the loss of cognitive function. That is clearly wrong under existing law. This point has enormous practical importance. The upper brain, which is the center of cognitive function, is more sensitive than the brainstem to interruptions in the oxygen supply (as may occur in a stroke or a near-drowning). It therefore often happens that the upper brain dies, or suffers permanent damage, while the brainstem remains relatively intact. The person then lapses into a coma, or vegetative state, in which all cognitive function is lost even though the brainstem functions and maintains respiration. If physicians believe the upper brain has really died, so that the condition is permanent, the patient will be diagnosed as being in a "permanent vegetative state" (PVS). Treatment decisions for patients in such a condition can present difficult ethical and legal problems, and these are addressed in the next Chapter. However, such patients are not dead. (Likewise, patients with an injury to the brain *stem* that is not fatal to that tissue—even though it may compromise spontaneous respiration or other vegetative functions—are not dead.).

Some have nonetheless advocated changing the law to replace whole brain death with *upper* brain death. The President's Commission and other authorities have rejected this position. One argument often offered for it is that personhood necessarily depends on the higher-brain functions of consciousness, rationality, and the capacity for mental or social functioning. But opponents point out that a cognition-based standard might result in defining newborns, or the severely mentally handicapped or demented, as dead, or at least not fully human. There is also doubt that we really would be willing to treat coma patients as dead. Would we be comfortable burying them without further ado, even while they are breathing? In sum, it is a serious business to label someone dead, and we are properly cautious in extending the definition.

Medical uncertainties would also arise in attempting such a definition. Even if we could determine precisely which portions of the brain house the cognitive functions essential to being called "alive" or a "person," we would sometimes have difficulty determining with sufficient certainty when, in fact, they have lost function irreversibly. See Chapter 7.D.2 (discussing the report of a woman who woke up from a 4–month coma, shortly after a judge ordered her feeding tubes removed); The Multi–Society Task Force on PVS, *Medical Aspects of the Persistent Vegetative State,* 330 New Eng. J. Med. 1572 (Second of Two Parts) (1994) (discussing prognosis of those in PVS of varying origins). Such errors are unavoidable, but we certainly want a definition that minimizes the frequency with which we mistakenly label someone dead.

In fairness, even the diagnosis of whole-brain death is not entirely without difficulty, since both expertise and technology are required. The influential "Harvard criteria" recommended in 1968 a series of diagnostic steps, including ruling out reversible causes (hypothermia, drug intoxification) and then finding, over a period of time, no response to painful stimuli, no spontaneous muscle movement, no reflexes, and a confirmatory "flat" electroencephalogram. These criteria have become generally accepted as establishing whole-brain death with adequate certainty. More updated guidelines for determining brain death have been published by various medical specialty societies.

Though the law is settled, a vigorous ethical and philosophical debate continues over the proper definition of death. In a society characterized by pluralistic religious and philosophical values, some have argued that we could plausibly leave it to individuals and their families to choose and apply their own definitions, perhaps within a range of acceptable predetermined alternatives (e.g., the three discussed above), or on the basis of a default rule that individuals would be free to alter within that same range. New Jersey law requires physicians to utilize cardiopulmonary criteria for determining death where there is reason to think that relying on neurological (brain) criteria will violate the decedent's religious beliefs. (The statute does not mention philosophical or secular beliefs as grounds for accommodation). This idea might be adopted to allow patients or families to elect *expanded* definitions of death based on their preferences or beliefs.

B. ORGAN PROCUREMENT AND ALLOCATION

This section explores, first, the basic legal rules governing how organs are obtained, and second, the system for the allocation of transplantable vital organs. The rules and policies governing both questions arise against the background reality that the need for vital organs persistently, and increasingly, exceeds their supply. In 1998, over 50,000 people were on organ transplant waiting lists. In 1996, a reported 4,022 people died while on such a list. (For related data, see http://www.unos.org). Even greater numbers of would-be transplantees never make it onto a waiting list (see sec. B.1., *infra*) since, due to the supply shortfall, it is clear from the outset they will not qualify.

This gap arises from many factors. On the supply side, people are hesitant, for many reasons, to fill out donor cards. After a death physicians may fail to ask family members for permission to harvest organs, and, if they do ask, will generally defer to any objections from anyone in the family, regardless of the deceased's wishes. Thus, although formal statements of a desire to donate one's organs upon death are *legally* controlling, Unif. Anatomical Gift Act § 2(h) (1987), these are routinely disregarded in favor of family members' views. On the demand side, while the number of transplants is growing, the waiting list is growing twice as fast. This may have to do with a simultaneous reduction in the number of medically suitable donors, through factors such as increased highway safety—seat belt laws, air bags, motorcycle helmets, enforcement of drunk driving laws—and an increase in the pool of potential recipients, through medical advances that render more people good candidates for transplantation.

1. Procurement of Organs

Laws and public polices that seek to procure more transplantable organs must balance the interests of donors, recipients, and the public health. In doing so, they confront two recurring dilemmas: the proper role of financial incentives in motivating donations, and the proper role of consent.

a. Organ Donation

Competent living persons may donate renewable tissues (blood, sperm) and those inessential to health (eggs), but not those necessary for sustaining their own life (liver, heart, both kidneys). While transplant centers will facilitate donation of a single kidney (or, less commonly, a lung, partial liver, or pancreas), particularly between family members, there are surgical as well as medical risks to the donor; life with a single kidney, for example, leaves the donor more vulnerable. There are also policy criticisms of this practice: within families there is a concern about coercion, and outside families, a concern about "under the table" payments. The latter implicates a federal prohibition of the *sale* of any transplantable organ (excluding blood, sperm or eggs), contained in the National Organ Transplant Act of 1984, 42 U.S.C. §§ 273–274g, which supplements traditional state-law regulation of the field.

Postmortem donations are governed by state law versions of the original (1968) or revised (1987) Uniform Anatomical Gift Act. Under these acts, which differ somewhat but have been adopted in some form in all states, competent adults may make gifts of their organs, effective at death, for education, research or transplantation. If a deceased person neither left instructions to make such a gift nor forbade it, his family may consent to organ harvesting. Under the revised (1987) version, hospitals are required not only to make routine inquiry of patients regarding their wish to be postmortem donors, but to ask families to exercise their authority to permit such donation (where the donor has not acted to prohibit this). The latter—"required request"—was designed to remedy physicians' reluctance to raise the question of donation with family members; it is also imposed on hospitals by federal law as a condition of participation in Medicare and Medicaid, 42 U.S.C. § 1320b–8. Required request has not, however, had much impact, since family members often refuse permission when asked. Like federal law, state law prohibits the sale of organs.

The legal prohibition against selling, during life, a vital organ whose removal is survivable (e.g., single kidney), *or* contracting for the sale of a heart, lungs, liver or both kidneys upon death, is justified on several theories. Its supporters argue that a market approach would "commodify" the body in objectionable ways, undermine altruism, and (in the context of organ removal during life) encourage needy persons to take inappropriate risks for pay. Advocates of a free market approach argue in response that the current system inhibits needed expansion in the supply of organs, and that it is unjust to donors since recipients, physicians and others all derive concrete benefits from the donors' largesse, yet donors remain uncompensated in material terms. Some observers have also noted that the donative element of the transaction creates complicated, enmeshing relationships—what has been called the "tyranny of the gift"—among the donee, the donor (if he is alive), and their respective families. Renee C. Fox & Judith Swazey, Spare Parts: Organ Replacement in American Society 40–41 (1992). The debate is ongoing, and merely summarized here.

b. *Donation and the Definition of Death*

More organs would be available for transplantation if the permanently unconscious were defined as dead (see § A.3, *supra*). Such an upper brain definition of death would include not only adults in a permanent coma but also anencephalic newborns, who are born with no upper brain. The argument for treating them as dead is especially strong since the complete absence of the upper brain removes any doubt about whether their condition is reversible. But the only case on point held that such a baby was not dead under state law, and therefore could not be used as a source of harvestable organs, as its parents had hoped. In re T.A.C.P., 609 So.2d 588 (Fla.1992).

Some suggest another halfway measure, short of full adoption of upper brain death: relax the "dead donor" requirement to allow organ harvesting from terminally ill or permanent coma patients who have specified, in an advance directive, that this is their wish. The problem is that since the patient is still alive under current law, removing an essential organ effectively constitutes murder—to which the victim's consent is no defense. The legal result is not altered by calling the procedure assisted suicide, as we see when that topic is explored in the next chapter. However, the potential to harvest more organs lends additional support to those who advocate legalizing voluntary euthanasia.

c. *Mandates and Novel Rules for Organ Procurement*

(1) *After Death.*

State law authorizes coroners or medical examiners to conduct autopsies for forensic or public health reasons, regardless of the family's wishes, or for other reasons if the family requests one. A number of state laws permit the removal of corneas from corpses during an autopsy, so long as there is no objection by the family. These laws, however, often impose no concomitant duty to notify the family or ascertain their views. Few families know they have the burden to object preemptively. Nevertheless, several courts have upheld constitutional challenges to such rules, relying on the state's interest in increasing the supply of useable corneas and the relatively limited nature of the bodily intrusion. One court, however, reasoned persuasively that the same state law that gives the family a right to object also confers on them a constitutionally cognizable "property" interest in the deceased's corneas, which carries with it some (unspecified) procedural due process protection. It is this procedural protection that is violated when a coroner fails to ascertain the family's wishes, even though there may be no substantive constitutional bar to the state more forthrightly allowing unconsented corneal harvesting. Brotherton v. Cleveland, 923 F.2d 477 (6th Cir.1991).

Several states (Texas, California, Maryland) authorize coroners to remove vital organs, rather than just corneas, though they require evidence that the decedent while alive did not object, and some efforts to contact the family. If contacted, the family can preclude harvesting; if not, coroners may proceed, but they may well be reluctant to do so. Unlike the corneal transplant laws, these laws are not widely used, nor has their constitutionality been tested on procedural or substantive grounds.

In connection with *either* corneas or vital organs, one might ask: if a policy of harvesting without affirmative objection or explicit consent is justified for autopsy cases (where there is already an established state interest in crime solving or in public health), could it properly be extended to *all* deaths, where the only state interest is in increasing the supply of organs? This is the "presumed consent" approach, advocated by some commentators and adopted in some European countries. It shifts the default position: all persons are *presumed* to have *consented* to organ harvesting unless they explicitly state otherwise. This approach has not been used or tested in the United States, and so it is not known whether it would overcome the noted tendency of physicians not to act without the family's permission. .

A final approach, somewhat less radical, is to require all individuals to make an explicit living choice about donation, at a designated time such as upon applying for a driver's license. Where "mandated choice" has been attempted, however, the refusal rate has remained quite high, perhaps because in the particular decisional settings little information has been provided.

(2) *During Life.*

Can organs not essential to a competent person's life ever be taken against his wishes? In the limited circumstances in which the question has arisen, the law has consistently prohibited such a step, even where the tissue is renewable and the procedure may be lifesaving. E.g., McFall v. Shimp, 10 Pa. D. & C3d 90 (1978) (discussed in Chapter 8.B.1). For an interesting argument defending the ethics of a law that would both compel everyone to be potential donors of renewable and non-essential tissues, and assure universal access to such tissues by all donees in need, see G. Calabresi, *Do We Own Our Bodies?*, 1 Health Matrix 5 (1991).

Difficult problems arise where the question is whether to allow organs to be taken from incompetent, living persons for the benefit of others, a situation in which the capacities to form a donative intent and to understand the procedure, as well as voluntariness, may all be lacking. There are two leading cases, with contrasting facts and results. Strunk v. Strunk, 445 S.W.2d 145 (Ky.1969), upheld an order authorizing a kidney transplant from a mentally retarded institutionalized man to his brother who was dying from kidney disease. No other family member had the requisite tissue compatibility, a cadaveric kidney apparently had not become available or was unsuitable, and the evidence indicated that the ward would be harmed less by the loss of a kidney than by the death of his brother, on whom he was quite emotionally dependent and who would be his caretaker after their parents died. In contrast, In re Pescinski, 226 N.W.2d 180 (Wis.1975), refused, ostensibly on jurisdictional grounds, to authorize transplant of a kidney from an institutionalized schizophrenic man to his sister for the same disease as in *Strunk*. Unlike *Strunk*, in *Pescinski* the incompetent donor's interests were not as strong: a competent brother was compatible but unwilling to donate, and the incompetent donor showed "marked indifference" to his environment, suggesting he had no real relationship with his siblings. Thus, there was no way to avoid the conclusion that an incompetent person was being exploited for another's benefit. Chapter 8.A.4 discusses similar concerns—complicated by the countervailing issues of parental and reproductive freedom—raised by reports of some parents who have conceived a child who, as an infant, can donate bone marrow to a sibling suffering from fatal anemia.

(3) *Ownership of Organs.*

Underlying many of these debates over organ procurement strategies are assumptions or disagreements over who, if anyone, "owns" organs and other body tissues, either during or after life. By "own," we mean any number of particular property-like interests or rights, including the right to control, consent, dispose of, and/or sell human tissues. Rather than declare any universal property status or immanent quality of human tissue, the law has reached a series of variable results based on particularized circumstances, informed by the value of a particular organ or tissue, the parties making claims upon it, and competing social interests. Space does not permit full discussion, but the range of possible results is suggested by the multiple opinions in the *Moore* case, discussed in Ch. 2.B.3.b, which posed ownership issues in a research, rather than a transplantation, context.

Moore held that a patient from whose tissues a commercial cell line was derived, without his knowledge or consent, had no tort claim for conversion, on the ground that he had no property interest in the cells once they were removed (with consent) from his body. (They came from a diseased spleen.) The majority was concerned that allowing a conversion action would unduly inhibit medical research.

A concurring justice found it ethically abhorrent to recognize human tissue as a commodity in which one has a financial interest. A concurrence/dissent argued that a conversion claim *could* lie under proper facts, noting that the law already recognizes property-like interests in controlling the disposition of one's organs. And a dissent argued strongly for immediate recognition of the conversion claim. As these opinions, and the divergent results in other settings, suggest, we are not likely to see a unified resolution of the ownership issue soon. Even less certain is how to resolve the futuristic debates, which are now at our doorstep, over ownership of new, bioengineered life forms.

2. Allocation of Organs

The National Organ Transplant Act of 1984 created the Organ Procurement and Transportation Network (OPTN), a private nonprofit entity, to oversee retrieval of organs and determine standards for their allocation. The United Network for Organ Sharing (UNOS) operates OPTN under contract with the Department of Health and Human Services (DHHS). UNOS is a membership organization that includes the country's 69 organ procurement organizations (OPOs), transplant centers, and others.

The first step to a needed transplant, from a patient's perspective, is getting on a waiting list. Once that occurs, the UNOS guidelines determine how OPOs allocate organs within their geographic area. We explore both steps.

a.   Waiting Lists and UNOS Distribution

A prospective donee's eligibility for a waiting list is determined locally, by individual transplant centers (generally located at select major hospitals), which develop and apply their own criteria. Scarcity requires rationing, and because failure to qualify at this critical first step effectively terminate's a candidate's eligibility, the stakes are very high. Many centers consider factors such as the prospects for successful surgery, the duration of the expected benefit, and the post-transplantation quality of life. Least controversial as bases for *excluding* candidates are medical considerations as to which there is some consensus, such as (in the case of a liver-transplant candidate) advanced heart or lung disease, or liver failure caused by Hepatitis B, which is likely to recur and infect the new liver.

Other factors, though, are more ethically complex. For example, in the case of liver transplants, centers vary on whether to list alcoholics and other substance abusers, whose habits may have caused their disease (and may threaten the new organ); the decision may turn on recent abstinence, stability, and other factors. Some assert that while alcoholics should not be given a lower priority because of *alcoholism*, they can be held to account for failure to obtain *treatment* that would forestall liver failure. Others think it is ill-advised to base standards on notions of individual responsibility due to inadequate consensus about virtue, undue selectivity about what behaviors will deserve eligibility, and unjustified invasions of privacy. Some centers exclude felony prisoners, or struggle with eligibility of those who have recently attempted suicide. In one recent case a 34–year old woman with Down Syndrome was rejected for a heart and lung transplant by the medical centers at Stanford University and UC–San Diego because physicians thought she was not sufficiently intelligent to comply with the complicated post-transplant drug regimen. Though both institutions eventually relented, the case illuminates the problems inherent in such criteria. Decisions are also influenced by ability to pay and the adequacy of insurance coverage.

In recent years, concerns have been voiced about the allocation system's overall fairness. The most serious arise from its "federated" nature: when an organ becomes available it is offered initially to qualifying, rank-ordered candidates in the *geographic area* from which the organ came; if it cannot be used there, it is then offered within the larger *region* (of which there are 11 nationwide); and only last is it offered nationally. Allocating organs *within* these sets of non-overlapping areas means that there can be significant differences in the waiting period—days to months, or more— *among* such areas, depending on supply and demand (and, sometimes, other factors). Regions with a sicker population, or whose medical centers attract more transplant referrals, have longer wait lists, and patients are free to shop the country for areas with shorter lists, which are often those with less established transplant centers. This partly explains why Mickey Mantle received a liver within a few days of acceptance on the waiting list, when the national average was two and half months.

These concerns, along with the view that technology has diminished the justifications for localized use first (e.g., time limits on the useful life of a harvested organ), have prompted DHHS to require more uniform medical criteria for wait list decisions and to more fully nationalize the organ distribution system. Various proposals are still being studied and debated. Critics respond, in general, that this initiative comes at the urging of the large, established transplant centers in order to increase the allocation of organs they receive from other regions of the country with shorter wait lists and smaller centers. The larger centers respond, in part, that they should receive more organs because their patients are more seriously ill and they typically have a better track record than less experienced transplant teams.

b.   *The Ethics of Allocation Policies*

Numerous organ allocation criteria are possible. "Social worth" is sometimes proposed, though it is widely rejected as unethical and unworkable in a pluralistic and humanistic society. Social worth may implicitly animate some decisions, however, perhaps in determining waiting list eligibility. Witness the following statement made by a lay member of one of the local committees assigned, in the 1960s, to allocate scarce kidney dialysis machines: "I remember voting against a young woman who was a known prostitute. I found I couldn't vote for her, rather than another candidate, a young wife and mother. I also voted against a young man who, until he learned he had renal failure, had been a ne'er-do-well, a real playboy." The comparative valuation of human lives is of course ethically unacceptable as a general proposition, but we may deceive ourselves if we think that all such distinctions can be avoided. For instance, they necessarily come into play to some extent in decisions about medical prognosis.

Even when criteria are unobjectionable in the abstract, they are difficult to apply, or rank order, in practice. Fairness or equality among candidates suggests relying on the length of time one has been on the waiting list, but this could give the organ to someone who has the least need. Maximizing the good that is done suggests giving organs to those who will live the longest, but this is in tension with another compelling principle known as the "rescue ethic," which is to avoid the most imminent harms. Being fair, doing good, and rescuing those in greatest peril are each valid principles, but they point to different patients, and people disagree on which should rank most highly. Therefore, present practice is to use a mixture of all three, with different weightings for different organs.

The OPOs, which are responsible for procuring organs in their region, make allocation decisions within regions based on uniform national policies promulgated by UNOS. While these policies differ as among particular organs, typical criteria, to which specified weights are attached for ranking purposes, include: the medical urgency of the donee's circumstances (this factor counts heavily in liver transplantation but is generally less critical for kidneys, where dialysis can often sustain the waiting donee); the likelihood of a successful transplant, including the expected length of the benefit (which in turn may depend, in part, on the donee's age and general health status, and on biological compatibility between donor and recipient—e.g., organ size, blood type, and genetic makeup); how long the candidate has been on the waiting list; and the candidate's ability to be transplanted immediately. For most organs, there is a point system that specifies how to weight each factor in a particular case to generate a final ranking.

As part of the current effort to more fully nationalize organ allocation, federal authorities recently required UNOS to adopt medical urgency as the cardinal standard, but this has engendered significant opposition, resulting in suspending the requirement pending further debate. A focus on medical urgency is subject to fair criticism for failing to derive the most benefit from a limited supply of organs, where benefit is measured not only by lives saved but also by total years of life preserved. A criterion of the sickest first can also serve as a proxy for allocating more organs to centers with longer wait lists, since patients' conditions tend to deteriorate over time. Whether, and in what form, the proposal will become law remains to be seen.

CHAPTER 7

THE LAW AND ETHICS OF WITH-HOLDING MEDICAL CARE AND ASSISTING SUICIDE

In earlier generations, most people died at home. Hospitals were not places to go for advanced medical treatment, because there was no advanced medical treatment. Hospitals were instead places that cared for people too poor or too alone for anyone to tend them properly at home. Changes in the function of the hospital began apace after World War II. In the last few decades especially, there has been a major social change in the expectations people have of medicine and doctors. Hospitals have become places where magic is done, where machines and procedures well beyond the ken of most people transform the sick and dying into—hopefully—the well and alive. Of course, even modern medicine cannot cure everyone. But the possibility requires the attempt.

The consequence is that most people now die in hospitals or nursing homes. The dying and the recovering share the technology, and often even the physicians cannot tell them apart. Perhaps another effort, another procedure, will change the illness' course. Processes designed to sustain life temporarily, until the body recovers, can continue it past all hope of recovery, so that death is prolonged rather than avoided. Families once had no control over the course of an illness, but great control over the environment in which it ran its course. Modern medicine often gives the physician hope to control the illness, but leaves the family feeling control over nothing. In this environment, the modern field of bioethics was born, with the realization that determining whether to employ the new medical tools is often a philosophical as well as a medical decision, requiring participation by the patient as well as the physician. The more recent advent of managed care suggests it is also an economic decision, with claims to input by the bill payer as well.

In re Quinlan, 355 A.2d 647 (N.J.1976) was the first well-known modern case to consider whether physicians may intentionally withdraw or withhold life-sustaining medical treatment from a seriously ill patient. Only 22, Karen Quinlan fell into a coma, or "persistent vegetative state," for reasons never established. She retained some brainstem function, and therefore was not brain dead, but the attending physicians believed she would never regain consciousness, and would soon die if they discontinued the use of a respirator to maintain her breathing. When the attending physician declined to follow her father's instructions to discontinue this life support, Joseph Quinlan sought a court order appointing him guardian of his adult daughter, with express authority to end "all extraordinary medical procedures." *Quinlan* held the father, along with Karen's physicians (whom as guardian he could appoint or dismiss) could withdraw the respirator after confirming Karen's gloomy prognosis with a hospital committee.

Fourteen years later very similar facts were presented in Cruzan v. Director, 497 U.S. 261 (1990). Nancy Cruzan's physicians placed a feeding tube down her throat when she lapsed into an unconscious state three weeks after suffering injuries in an automobile accident. But later they also concluded that their patient was in a persistent vegetative state. When hospital personnel refused to honor their request to withdraw the artificially provided nutrition and hydration, Nancy's parents obtained a trial court order that they do so. But the Missouri Supreme Court reversed, concluding that state law did not give the parents authority to make this decision without clear and convincing evidence that Nancy would have agreed. The U.S. Supreme Court held that Missouri's evidentiary requirement did not violate the Constitution. Some issues common to *Quinlan* and *Cruzan* reappear throughout this chapter:

1. If we know the patient's views about her medical care, must we necessarily follow them? Might we decline when a patient refuses food or water? Artificially supplied food or water? When a patient asks for medication or procedures that have no purpose other than hastening her death?

2. If the patient's views govern, what evidence do we need to establish what it is? Karen Quinlan

and Nancy Cruzan could not themselves instruct their physicians. There was testimony that Karen had expressed, in social conversations, a distaste for heroic medical measures. Are such reports adequate to establish what she would now want done? Do even fully documented advance directives deserve the same deference as the patient's contemporaneous instructions?

3. Who speaks on behalf of a patient who leaves no advance directive. Is a family relationship sufficient to confer authority, or is a court appointment needed? What standard is appropriate to guide the decisionmaker's judgment?

4. Does it matter, ethically or legally, whether the proposed decision would a) discontinue treatment that has been ongoing, as opposed to withholding a new therapy; b) actively withdraw a treatment, as by disconnecting a respirator, in contrast with not acting, as by failing to provide the next dose of an essential medication? Is there any meaning of moral significance to the question of whether a treatment is "ordinary" or "extraordinary"?

We consider each of these issues, and others as well. We begin by examining the traditional ethical distinctions that focus on the nature of the act by which treatment is ended, or on the nature of the treatment; we then go on to survey the modern analysis based on the competing principles of patient autonomy and medical paternalism.

A. THE TRADITIONAL ETHICAL DISTINCTIONS

1. Acting Versus Failing to Act

There is a long moral and legal tradition, developed independently of medical ethics, distinguishing culpability for positive acts from culpability for failing to act. In this larger context the distinction has great importance. For example, traditional common law doctrine creates no general duty to rescue, so that while one is clearly liable, both civilly and criminally, for pushing another into turbulent waters, one is not liable for failing to rescue a drowning stranger. By analogy, one might thus expect that non-treatment decisions implemented by a positive act would be more problematic than those in which the physician simply does not administer a potential therapy. The act/non-act distinction of the common law does not apply so easily, however, to medical care decisions. The traditional common law rule has well established exceptions, under which an affirmative duty to act does arise in some cases, as a result of the relationship between the parties. For example, a parent, or even a third party who is acting in the parent's place, may have a duty to act to rescue their child, where the rescue does not place an undue risk on the caretaker. When a child falls off a playground swing and lies injured on the ground, the accompanying parent or teacher cannot rely on the general common law rule to escape liability for failing to come to the child's assistance. The attending physician caring for a hospital patient has a similar obligation, thus creating a duty to act in some cases.

Barber v. Superior Ct., 195 Cal.Rptr. 484 (App. 1983) made this point in the context of an indictment for murder brought against attending physicians who had honored the family's request to withdraw a comatose patient's respirator and intravenous feeding and hydration tubes. The court held that the indictment should be dismissed after finding that the withdrawn treatment was "ineffective," and that physicians have no affirmative duty to provide ineffective treatment to their patients. Had the court concluded that the treatment in question was "effective," then the physicians would have been under an affirmative duty to provide it and criminal liability might have resulted. *Barber* illustrates that physicians can be liable for a failure to act, depending upon later evaluations of the appropriateness of the omitted treatment. The utility of the act/non-act distinction is thus largely eliminated.

Barber also illustrates another difficulty with the application of the "act/omission" distinction to treatment termination cases, for the case actually involved an act rather than an omission, despite the court's conclusion to the contrary. The physicians in *Barber* removed the patient's respirator in the expectation that his death would soon result; when it did not, after two days, they removed the feeding and hydration tubes. There can be no question that under the act/omission distinction as understood in the common law generally, the physicians "acted" when they removed the tubes, just as a bystander would have acted in pulling a life preserver out of a drowning man's reach. The bystander has no duty to throw the life preserver to the desperate swimmer in the first instance, but he cannot rely on that principle to avoid liability for removing it. Similarly, the act/omission distinction cannot exculpate a physician who removes a respirator, even if he had no duty initially to provide it. Thus if the *Barber* court was ethically correct in dismissing the indictment, as almost all agree, the act/omission distinction does not explain why.

We can now see that in some cases (like *Barber*) we will wish to avoid liability even though there has been an affirmative act, while in other cases a physician will be under a duty to act and therefore liable even for an omission. The effort to sort termination of treatment cases according to whether they involve "acting" or "failing to act" thus confuses rather than assists the legal and ethical analysis. This does not prevent courts and commentators from continuing to rely upon it, however. See the discussion below of active versus passive euthanasia.

2. Withholding Versus Withdrawing Treatment

In referring to acts and omissions, the *Barber* court may well have had a different but related distinction in mind. Courts and commentators sometimes distinguish between "withdrawing" treatment, which they then assume to be wrong, and "withholding" treatment, which may be permissible. Observers sometimes assume that withdrawal of treatment necessarily involves an act rather than an omission, while withholding treatment is assumed to be an omission. This is incorrect, however.

For example, a physician might prescribe a course of antibiotics whose effectiveness requires uninterrupted treatment over a week. If one stops providing the pills after two days, one is "withdrawing" the treatment, although the withdrawal is carried out by an omission rather than by an act. The court in *Barber* relied upon just such reasoning in asserting that the withdrawal of hydration was an omission. In that case, of course, hydration was provided technologically, and withdrawal was carried out by an act disconnecting the apparatus that would otherwise continue to hydrate the patient automatically. But since other treatments are not provided automatically, and their discontinuance requires only an omission rather than an act, the court chose to treat this withdrawal of hydration as an omission as well. While this reasoning is surely specious—the fact that some other treatment could be withdrawn by an omission hardly converts the act in *Barber* into a nonact—it does illustrate judicial acceptance of the fact that "withdrawal" and "act" are not coextensive categories.

Nor is it clear that every case of withholding treatment involves an omission rather than an act, although this will usually be the case. Consider, however, a nurse who is about to insert a respirator in the patient, when an attending physician intervenes and keeps her from doing so. This sequence is not distinguishable from the case in which a bystander is about to throw a life preserver to a drowning man, when a second bystander intervenes to keep him from doing so. The second bystander might have a right to intervene—perhaps she owns the life preserver, is about to leave, and wishes to take it with her. But whether or not her acts are justifiable, they are acts and not omissions. The same is true of the intervening physician, who has acted to withhold a treatment.

It is thus clear that if the "withdraw/withhold" distinction has any utility at all, it derives from some independent principle, and not from any similarity we may have thought it had to the distinction between acting and omitting. In fact, the withdraw/withhold distinction is if anything even worse than that between acting and omitting to act, which may at least be helpful in contexts other than medical decisionmaking. The distinction between withholding and withdrawing treatment has no other arena in which it can offer insight, and it certainly offers little to medical decisionmaking.

Those who seek to rely on the distinction typically assume that withholding treatment, like omitting to act, is somehow more defensible than withdrawing treatment. Yet clearly, withholding treatment cannot be generally permissible: it is the essence of the physician's and hospital's obligation to *provide* beneficial therapy to their patients. Justification for withholding treatment in particular cases must thus rely on a special feature of those cases rather than on the fact that treatment was withheld. But it is not clear that any such features, when present, would justify the withholding of treatment but not its withdrawal. In fact, many if not most modern cases concluding that treatment may be terminated involve the authorization of withdrawal rather than withholding, for the simple reason that the life sustaining treatment which is the subject of the decision had already been begun, so that any action necessarily involves its withdrawal. The most common and obvious example is the withdrawal of the ventilator in cases like *Quinlan* and *Barber*.

Moreover, as was pointed out by the President's Commission for the Study of Ethical Problems in Medicine and Biomedical and Behavioral Research, in their volume Deciding to Forego Life Sustaining Treatment, reliance on the distinction between withholding and withdrawing easily produces pernicious consequences. On one hand, we might end up continuing a treatment long after it is on balance beneficial for the patient, on the mistaken grounds that discontinuance requires some special justification. And perhaps even more troubling, we may resist starting a therapy that has some chance of improving health or prolonging life because of our fear that we may be unable to stop it, even if it proves less beneficial than we had hoped.

3. Active and Passive Euthanasia

"Euthanasia," or mercy killing, are emotional terms, the use of which usually shed more heat than light. That is in part because the terms communicate the proponent's concession that the actor intends to cause the victim's death, albeit with the justification that the killing is motivated by compassion for the victim, not animus. Because euthanasia has historically been condemned both legally and morally, legally accepted decisions to terminate medical care are not ordinarily described as euthanasia even when they fit the definition. The historical condemnation of euthanasia is influenced heavily by fears, born of actual experience, that its acceptance leads too easily to the cynical and evil-intentioned killings of the vulnerable and helpless under its rubric. The mass slaughter of the mentally ill and developmentally disabled by the Nazi government is perhaps the most often cited example.

In light of this history it is not surprising that courts, legislatures, and commentators sometimes engage in rather transparent self-deception in order to distinguish a withdrawal of care, which they would allow, from improper "euthanasia." Typical is California's Natural Death Act, whose very purpose is to provide a means for individuals to leave instructions (through "living wills") for shortening their life by withholding medical care in specified circumstances, but which nonetheless specifies that it does not "condone, authorize, or approve mercy killing or assisted suicide or permit any affirmative or deliberate act or omission to end life other than to permit the natural process of dying." California Health and Safety Code § 7191.5. The statutory distinction, occasionally found also in the cases, is

312 THE RIGHT TO DIE Ch. 7

between causing death by the withdrawal of care rather than by "natural" processes, which by definition does not constitute mercy killing. Such an argument relies on an unusual conception of cause which the law would not normally accept.

The flaw in this view of causation can be seen most easily by imagining the removal of a ventilator from a seriously ill patient unable to breathe without it, an act the statute intends to authorize in specified circumstances. If the ventilator is withdrawn by a physician acting pursuant to the directions of the living will, we are apparently to conclude that nothing has happened but "the natural process of dying." Suppose, however, that the same ventilator were removed instead by the patient's nephew, who hoped thereby to advance the date of his inheritance. He can and should be charged with murder. Can he plead in defense that he did not cause his Uncle's death, which was merely the outcome of "the natural process of dying"? Hardly. Our intuition, of course, is that the two cases are different, and surely they are. But the reason cannot be that in one case removal of the ventilator was the cause of death, and in the other it was not. Both expected death to result from their act and both were right. Under ordinary legal usage, therefore, not only did both cause the death, but both *intended* it.

The only apparent difference between the two cases is the motivation of the actor, their *reason* for removing the ventilator and intending the patient's death. One acts from selfish motivation, the other out of compassion. But of course that difference defines the classic understanding of euthanasia: mercy killing. If we accept that difference as the explanation of why one act is justified and the other is not, we thereby accept the basic premise upon which the legalization of euthanasia is urged. No American legislature or court has yet confronted and accepted this reality directly, although the result in most of the recent cases cannot otherwise be explained.

One halfway measure would rely upon the distinction between active and passive euthanasia. As these terms are commonly used, mercy killing is acceptable only if it is passive; active killing is never justified regardless of its motivation. Obviously, this distinction is largely a replay of the distinction between acting and failing to act, although it not entirely the same since in the medical context passive euthanasia is usually meant to encompass any intentional non-treatment, whether achieved by a withholding or withdrawal of care, and whether it involves an act or a failure to act. The withdrawal of a respirator or the failure to provide needed antibiotics would thus both be passive euthanasia, if motivated by mercy for the patient; the injection of a lethal dose of morphine to the terminal patient in great pain would be active euthanasia and thus not permitted under this analysis.

This distinction between active and passive euthanasia is defended largely on pragmatic grounds: it erects a plateau in the slippery slope otherwise created by accepting euthanasia. A general acceptance of euthanasia would mean that we would be left to distinguish justified from unjustified killing entirely in terms of the actor's motive, and most think that assessments of such a subjective state cannot establish a sufficiently bright line, given what would be at stake. But the problem seems more manageable if we open the door to passive euthanasia only. Most examples of unacceptable killings masquerading as euthanasia involve active rather than passive measures. The murderer motivated by something other than mercy cannot usually wait for his intended victim to require some life sustaining measure that he then can fail to provide. In our everyday experience there is a correlation between motive and the active or passive nature of conduct—active killing is rarely motivated by mercy; letting die may well be. If allowing passive euthanasia will risk only a few scattered cases of wrongful killing, we may be more willing to rely on our ability to assess motive to sort which cases are authorized and which are prohibited.

This analysis, unfortunately, may have less utility in the medical context than it does generally. First, as we have already observed, physicians are under a duty to provide beneficial treatment to their patients, and their omissions are much more likely to be culpable. In addition, our everyday experience may not translate properly into the hospital context. While most individuals rarely have the opportunity to bring about another's death through an omission rather than an act, hospital personnel often do. There are thus differences both in duty and in opportunity that may reduce, in the medical context, the pragmatic advantage the distinction may otherwise offer in mitigating the problem of the slippery slope. If one in fact believes that motive is a dangerously ephemeral basis upon which to distinguish justified from unjustified killings, then one may well wish to reject passive as well as active euthanasia.[1]

Not only may unacceptable dangers lurk in allowing passive euthanasia, but at the same time, an inflexible rule limiting euthanasia to passive measures may prove unacceptable. A proposal to allow passive but not active euthanasia must assume that in the small group of cases in which we wish to allow euthanasia, we will usually have the opportunity to bring it about humanely by terminating treatment. So if the doctor's justified merciful intentions can be carried out by declining to provide intravenous fluids, there is surely no need to risk moral confusion between this case and another by allowing him to shoot the patient instead. This is probably right as far as it goes: where suitable passive measures are available, we should employ them alone. The problem is that they will not always be available, and some of the cases in which they will not be available are among the most compelling for allowing euthanasia. The classic case is the terminal cancer patient in overwhelming pain. Sufficiently large doses morphine might relieve his pain, but those same doses will shorten his life by depressing his respiration. Sometimes there is no dosage adequate to relieve the pain that will

1.   The problem is not entirely theoretical, as shown by these newspaper articles. "Killing of 49 Elderly Patients By Nurse Aides Stun Austria," New York Times, April 18, 1989, at A1; "Former Nurse's Aide Pleads Guilty In Murders of At Least 24

not lead almost immediately to his death, especially given the patient's already weakened condition. If we wait long enough we will undoubtedly have the opportunity to allow the patient to die, but in the intervening days or weeks the patient will continue to suffer horribly. Relieving this patient's pain thus requires active euthanasia.

There is currently no legal authority that generally justifies active euthanasia. Even Oregon's much debated legalization of assisted suicide, discussed further in section C.4, is limited in several important ways. For example, a physician may prescribe but not administer a lethal medication. Yet throughout the country physicians have often provided terminal patients in terrible pain with life-shortening doses of morphine, and prosecutions for such conduct are essentially unheard of. A concurring judge in Bouvia v. Superior Court of Los Angeles County, 225 Cal.Rptr. 297 (Cal.App.1986), described more fully below, perhaps responding to this dilemma, urged that the law recognize a "right to die" that would include the right "to enlist assistance from others, including the medical profession, in making death as painless and quick as possible."

4. The Doctrine of Double Effect

Those who ordinarily oppose active euthanasia sometimes try to explain their willingness to allow a morphine injection in this case by reference to what is called "the doctrine of double effect." The idea is that the physician intends only to relieve the patient's pain; while morphine will also kill the pa-

in Ohio," New York Times, August 19, 1987, at A1; "Patient Testifies Against His Nurse," New York Times, October 7, 1984, at A16.

tient this second effect is not intended, and the physician's act is therefore not wrong. The problem is that the doctrine serves only to excuse the ignorant. The ordinarily competent physician who is aware of morphine's full effect can hardly escape responsibility by saying that he did not intend the death that he knew would result from his act. The law generally assumes that people intend the ordinary and foreseeable consequences of their acts, and acceptance of this defense would therefore require employing a new and special definition of "intent." It is more accurate to say that the physician's *motive* for administering the morphine is to relieve pain and not to kill, but once again, to accept this distinction is merely to agree that killing motivated by compassion is acceptable, a proposition which would justify euthanasia generally.

5. Ordinary Versus Extraordinary Treatment

In discussions of treatment termination cases one often hears a distinction made between ordinary and extraordinary treatment. The thought is that while physicians have a duty to provide ordinary treatment, they have no duty to provide extraordinary treatment. The same thought may be put other ways as well. One might hear the view that in not providing "extraordinary" treatment one is merely letting "nature take its course." As with the other rules of thumb offered to resolve treatment termination cases, this one does not bear up well under examination. As the *Quinlan* court lamented in trying to make sense of this approach, "the record here is somewhat hazy in distinguishing between ordinary and extraordinary measures."

The distinction between ordinary and extraordinary treatment has its most important source in Roman Catholic theology, and has been the subject of statements by two Popes. But as Paul Ramsey observed in *The Patient as Person,* physicians, as well as many laymen, often use these terms differently than do Popes and philosophers. Physicians may assume that ordinary is synonymous with "customary," and that extraordinary treatment is therefore simply treatment that goes beyond that which is usually provided. Some reflection reveals, however, that these definitions cannot offer much assistance in thinking through the ethical issues. If we conclude that a respirator is ordinary treatment, then we could not remove it from Karen Ann Quinlan. But if we conclude that it is extraordinary, and believe that this distinction explains what we can and cannot do, it would seem that we could withdraw the respirator from a patient recovering from surgery, as well as from Karen Quinlan. This surely won't do. As the *Quinlan* court itself observed, one must then conclude that the same respirator is extraordinary in some cases but ordinary in others. The distinction then, if it is to make any ethical sense, cannot depend upon any quality inherent in the treatment itself, but must rather appeal to the larger context in which the treatment is provided.

This understanding of the distinction is expressed in the standard definition provided by Ramsey. "*Ordinary* means of preserving life are all medicines, treatments and operations which offer a reasonable hope of benefit for the patient and which can be obtained and used without excessive expense, pain, or other inconvenience.... Extraordinary means of preserving life ... mean all medicines, treatments, and operations, which cannot be obtained without excessive expense, pain or other inconvenience, or which, if used, would not offer a reasonable hope of benefit." It thus becomes clear that the same treatment can be ordinary in one case and extraordinary in another.

Yet while this standard definition shows how the distinction can be ethically relevant, it is more a label than an explanation because it avoids confronting the key questions. What kinds of benefits are adequate to justify requiring continued treatment? What is our standard for determining the kind of pain or expense that is so "excessive" as to render a treatment extraordinary, even if it would provide benefit? The definitions hedge even the most fundamental questions. For example, do we consider only the patient's "expense" or "inconvenience," or can we conclude that a treatment is extraordinary because of the inconvenience it imposes on other people? In a 1957 statement the Pope described "ordinary" means as "means that do not involve any grave burden for oneself or another." Later Papal statements, in 1958 and 1980, indicate that treatment can be ended if it imposes excessive burdens on the family, or if "the investment in instruments or personnel is disproportionate to the results foreseen." Others would insist that only the patient's own interests can be taken into account in deciding whether treatment should be ended. There is obviously nothing in the labels "ordinary" and "extraordinary" that can help resolve that debate. As was concluded by the President's Commission for the Study of Ethical Problems in Medicine and Biomedical and Behavioral Research, in its volume *Deciding to Forego Life–Sustaining Treatment* 88 (1983), the words function more as conclusory labels than as aids to ethical analysis.

6. Conclusion

The preceding sections have exposed the flaws in some commonly offered distinctions, but our appreciation of those flaws need not lead us to conclude that all acts or omissions that bring about a patient's death are wrong, or that courts would or should normally impose liability upon the physicians in all such cases. To the contrary, we have already noted the dismissal of the indictment in *Barber* and the authorization of the removal of the respirator in *Quinlan,* and we will see that these decisions are typical. But by first clearing away some common but ultimately unhelpful explanations for these results, we will better understand the proper basis for them.

In fact, in many cases motive may well be the only difference between proper termination of medical care and conduct which we want to condemn as murder. But as we have already noted, motive is for most courts and commentators an inadequate basis upon which to authorize life-ending acts. Legislatures and courts committed to not recognizing euthanasia cannot proceed with distinctions based entirely on motive. That realization has pushed both courts and ethicists to rely on an entirely different principle in these cases: the principle of personal autonomy. It is that to which we now turn.

B. THE COMPETING PRINCIPLES OF PERSONAL AUTONOMY AND BENEFICENCE

Coloring almost all debates over the appropriate decisions in termination of care cases is the principle of personal autonomy: the belief that each individual has the right to make decisions as to matters that primarily affect himself. Personal autonomy is an extraordinarily powerful principle in the modern western democracy. It is foundational to our political thinking; the vindication of personal autonomy is one of the primary aspects of the historical movement from Kings and dictators to constitutional democracies. It lies at the heart of many American constitutional principles. "The only purpose for which power can be rightfully exercised over any member of a civilized community, against his will, is to prevent harm to others. His own good, either physical or moral, is not a sufficient warrant." John Stuart Mill's views, expressed in *On Liberty* in 1859, strike most modern Americans as essentially correct, even if they appreciate that governance is necessarily a bit more complicated than that. Our belief in the importance of personal autonomy is now almost instinctual. Since we start from such strongly held commitments, it is hardly surprising that most people think it self-evident that no one may be compelled to submit to medical treatment against his will, at least if he is a competent adult deciding for himself. Nor is it surprising that most courts will seek to find, in the autonomy principle, warrant for their decisions on the termination of care.

The principle of personal autonomy is of course most obviously relevant to the case of an alert, competent adult capable of expressing his or her view at the time of the treatment decision. But it may be relied upon in other cases as well, and often is. There is the person who is not now competent or capable of expressing his view, but who left instructions when he was, that arguably apply now. There is the person who appointed a spokesman when competent, to decide for her if she were later unable to express her views. There is the spokesman appointed or assumed by law, such as the appointed guardian or the natural parent. Does the principle of personal autonomy apply in such cases as well? We will consider each of these cases in turn. For each we will discover that there is a competing principle that gradually increases in importance as we find reliance on autonomy more attenuated: the principle of beneficence, or doing good. Mill may have believed that power cannot be exercised for the good of the subject, but most people in fact accept some paternalism as necessary, and in some cases, perhaps even ethically compelled.

This conflict between autonomy and beneficence is particularly important in medicine. Physicians are experts, people who are consulted because they know more than lay people about the problem at hand. We consult experts not just for the information they can provide but also for their judgments. Lawyers, for example, often make decisions for their clients in part because the client *wants* to be instructed on what to do. The professional culture of medicine, into which physicians are trained, is even more steeped in paternalism. Physicians, unlike attorneys, do not typically think of themselves as their patient's agent. Agents are subject to the instructions of their principal in a way that physicians are not accustomed to. The strong paternalistic tradition in medicine has often been seen in discussions of the doctrine of informed consent. Even the most patient oriented versions of the modern doctrine, represented by the well-known case of Canterbury v. Spence, 464 F.2d 772 (D.C.Cir.1972), accept the need to leave some room for the case, however rare, in which the physician reasonably decides that the patient's interests require nondisclosure of material information. In other words, the very legal doctrine that emerges from, and has the very purpose of protecting, the patient's autonomy—the doctrine of informed consent—recognizes the need to limit that autonomy by leaving some role for physician paternalism.

Nonetheless, the most influential modern cases concerning the withdrawal or withholding of care rely heavily on the doctrine of personal autonomy.

Modern cases deal with variations on two main problems: Are there any limits appropriately put on the deference we pay a competent patient's choices about himself, when those choices are clear? And what does the autonomy principle tell us when the patient's views are obscure or inaccessible at the time of decision? The cases are conveniently placed in three categories: the currently competent patient, the formerly competent patient, and the never-competent patient. We consider each in turn.

C. THE CURRENTLY COMPETENT PATIENT

1. Paternalism and the Limits of Autonomy

Do the expressed wishes of a competent patient concerning her medical treatment, communicated at the time of decision, trump all competing concerns? Or are there limits to autonomy even here? Consider that many states continue to criminalize attempted suicide, and that all states retain general prohibitions on aiding and abetting the suicide of another. We consider below (section C.4) recent efforts to permit a limited form of assisted suicide for some terminally ill patients, but note that even these most far reaching proposals do not embrace the principle that people are entitled to enlist others to assist them in taking their own lives for any reason they deem sufficient. The significance of society's resistance to embracing any such general right is obscured in the medical context, because the cases put within that framework usually involve patients who want to die for reasons that many observers find sufficient. Yet to honor the principle of autonomy, without limit, is to believe the reasons are not relevant—that the decision, being entirely the patient's, is unreviewable by others. That extreme view cannot be reconciled with a legal system that retains any limitations on suicide. We consider here why we might want to retain some limits, even in the medical context.

Consider an otherwise healthy patient who is hospitalized from injuries incurred in a failed suicide attempt. The patient contracts an infection, easily treatable with antibiotics but otherwise fatal. Few would suggest that a physician must yield without question to the patient's request that antibiotics be withdrawn. Or consider a patient just abandoned by his spouse, exacerbating the ordinary depression brought on by serious illness. Shall a physician simply accept the patient's decision to decline routine treatment that would restore health? If the medical opportunity had not presented itself, the same person who now seeks the physician's cooperation might have sought their neighbor's instead. But even the staunchest "right to die" advocate is unlikely to believe himself justified in expeditiously shooting anyone who asks to be killed, without further inquiry. If the neighbor should make an inquiry before acting, then so should the physician. Even if we believe suicide is justified in many cases, we must also concede that a e physician asked to forego life-sustaining treatment is morally obliged to exercise some independent judgment before honoring the request. In short, an element of beneficence—of paternalism—always limits the scope of autonomy. To concede that, of course, is not to establish the proper scope of paternalism, as to which there will be wide disagreement. But it should be clear at least that the autonomy principle cannot trump all other concerns, even though it is a powerful factor.

2. Determining Decisionmaking Capacity

The student committed to autonomy may be tempted at this point to suggest that the only inquiry that the physician or neighbor must make in the situations just described is one of competence: We must pause only to assure ourselves that the patient has the mental capacity to make the decision; once so assured we must then apply the autonomy principle and defer to the patient's wishes. Whatever the merits of that view in the abstract, it fails as a practical test of how to proceed because there is no generally accepted unitary standard of the requisite mental capacity to make medical decisions. Some people—the severely retarded or comatose—may be incompetent for all purposes, so that all would agree that we can never rely on their judgments in making medical decisions for them. But other cases are more difficult. There is in fact no bright line separating the competent from the incompetent, as mental capacity varies along a continuum.

The Hastings Center Guidelines on the Termination of Life Sustaining Treatment suggest distinguishing between "incompetence" and "incapacity." They would restrict use of the term "incompetent" to situations in which a formal judicial finding has been made that a person cannot make legally effective decisions as to their own affairs. They point out that persons who are legally competent may nonetheless lack the capacity to make a particular treatment decision, while persons who have been declared incompetent for certain purposes, such as managing their financial affairs, may nonetheless have sufficient capacity to make a treatment decision. The President's Commission, in its volume *Making Health Care Decisions,* concludes that the presence or absence of adequate decisionmaking capacity must be assessed in relation to the specific decision to be made, and not by global assessments of the person. The President's Commission therefore shares the view that a legal judgment (in either direction) of whether a person is competent to manage their financial affairs or the logistics of daily living is not necessarily dispositive on the separate question of whether a person has the capacity to make a particular health care decision.

How then is capacity to make health care decisions to be judged? Decisions based entirely on a person's status (child/adult; mentally retarded/mentally normal) are inconsistent with the approach favored by the Hastings Center and the President's Commission. Instead, both would employ what Hastings calls a "process" standard—an assessment in each case of whether the patient has the abilities necessary to make the particular decision at hand. Both agree that making such decisions requires a) possession of a set of values and goals, b) the ability to understand the facts relevant to the decision, c) the ability to reason about the decision, and d) the ability to communicate the decision. Of course, assessing whether a particular patient has the requisite decisionmaking capacity for the particular decision at hand will not always be easy. But this analysis does help avoid some common mistakes. First, we can see that the patient's expression of a preference does not alone establish the requisite decisionmaking capacity, since the ability to communicate a preference is only one of the necessary elements. Second, the patient's capacity is not appropriately judged by reference solely to the content of the patient's decision. We cannot conclude that a patient lacks the necessary decisionmaking capacity solely because the attending physicians believe that the patient's decision is "wrong" or "irrational."

At the same time, it is clear that the content of a patient's decision must influence the assessment of capacity. At a practical level, it is inevitable that patient decisions which their doctors and family view as reasonable will rarely if ever be challenged for incapacity. Not all decisions others see as unreasonable will be challenged, but they are the only decisions others are likely to scrutinize with care. But even at a level of principle, the content of the decision cannot be entirely irrelevant. Especially because judgments of capacity will be uncertain in some cases, it becomes important to determine how certain we must be of the patient's capacity before according their view the substantial weight required by the principle of autonomy. The choice, as noted by Buchanan and Brock, *Deciding for Others*, 64 Milbank Quarterly 17, 30 (Supp. 2, 1986), involves balancing the risk of denying the patient's self-determination (autonomy) against the risk of failing to protect from harm a patient unable to protect himself (beneficience and paternalism). As we raise the standard for decisionmaking capacity, we heighten the chance of the first error and lower the chance of the second. Our standard of decisionmaking capacity must thus reflect the relative weight we accord these two principles. On this question, the Commission plausibly concluded that we may demand more evidence of the patient's decisionmaking capacity as the consequences of following the patient's expressed preference become more substantial. In short, the greatest confidence is required before acting on a decision that will end the patient's life.

This discussion of capacity thus tells us that at a minimum, a physician is justified, and probably obliged, to refuse to act immediately on a patient's request to discontinue life-sustaining treatment, despite the importance of patient autonomy. Seriously ill people often suffer transitory depression. Patients who feel very bad often doubt any assurance that they will eventually feel better, whatever logical and factual basis the doctor might offer for his hopeful prediction. Physicians are familiar with the pattern of the depressed patient who is later grateful that the physician kept treating despite the patient's earlier indifference or resistance. We might say that when ill such a patient temporarily lacked the capacity to understand relevant facts or to reason from them. Yet some of these patients seem lucid and rational by ordinary standards—far above the line a court would require before judging them "incompetent." And indeed, decisionmaking capacity may not be the issue at all. Illness may affect a patient's decisions about her medical care by rendering temporary changes in her values rather than her capacity. Perhaps the depressed patient is unable to tolerate uncertainty in the healing process that he would ordinarily accept, and therefore demands more assurance than he would usually need or that medicine can usually provide.

Such possibilities suggest it is advisable to test the *durability* of the patient's decision (and thus his new values) before acting, when the consequences of acting are significant. When a doctor delays acting to test whether the patient's current decision is driven by a temporary set of values, the doctor acts both from paternalistic motivations, relying on the principle of beneficence, and in the belief that the patient will eventually agree that continuing treatment is in his interest. (One may say that the physician's act is also respectful of patient autonomy, if one believes the autonomy principle requires deference to the patient's long term values, rather than his current ones—and if the physician proves correct in her scepticism of the durability of the patient's current view.) Such acts by physicians are not uncommon, and therefore provide an important example of one way in which medicine routinely and correctly limits the scope of autonomy in dealing with patients who possess decisionmaking capacity.

3. Examples of Decisionmaking With the Competent Patient

Satz v. Perlmutter, 362 So.2d 160 (Fla.App.), aff'd, 379 So.2d 359 (1980), involved a 73 year old patient with Lou Gehrig's disease, which had progressed to the point of fairly general paralysis. He remained "in command of his faculties" and could still speak with great effort, although he required mechanical assistance to breathe. He would die soon regardless of what was done for him, but he had decided that he wanted the respirator removed from his trachea. Such removal would cause his death within one hour, according to the attending physicians. He had attempted to remove it himself and succeeded on at least one occasion; hospital personnel, alerted by an alarm connected to the respirator, had reattached it. His family supported his decision to remove it. The hospital declined to honor his request, largely out of fear of both criminal and civil liability, a fear which the court conceded "cannot be discounted." Abe Perlmutter, the patient, therefore petitioned the court for an order restraining hospital personnel from interfering with his decision to have the respirator removed. The state intervened in opposition to the petition, arguing that it had an overriding duty to preserve life and that termination of the "supportive care" would constitute an unlawful killing under state law. The trial court granted Perlmutter's petition, and was affirmed.

Perlmutter is a classic case for application of the autonomy principle, its essential facts repeated often in the modern hospital. The terminally ill patient who will die soon in any event asks to end the waiting because he finds his condition intolerable. Abe Perlmutter told the trial judge that whatever the consequence if the respirator were removed, "it can't be worse than what I am going through now." Most people find Perlmutter's decision entirely reasonable, whatever they would do themselves. So we have no reason to doubt Perlmutter's capacity and no paternalistic motivation to override his choice. Even the hospital probably agreed. It resisted only from fear of liability, which the court could put to rest.

Compare McKay v. Bergstedt, 801 P.2d 617 (Nev. 1990). Kenneth had been a quadriplegic since a swimming pool accident at the age of ten. He nonetheless completed high school. Now 31, he wrote poetry on a computer, read and watched television. Although permanently dependent upon a respirator, his condition was not terminal. But he wanted to die. He had been dependent upon his parents since his accident, but his mother had died and his father was fatally ill with lung cancer. He lived in terror that after his father's death a mishap would occur with his respirator which no one would be there to fix, leaving him to a horrible death. He sought a court order permitting the removal of his respirator by someone who could also deliver a sedative, granting legal immunity to the person providing that assistance, and absolving him of suicide for seeking this arrangement. He prevailed in both the trial court and state supreme court (whose decision was rendered after his death), the state offering only token opposition.

Kenneth presents a more difficult case than does Abe Perlmutter. Abe was on the verge of death in any event, while Kenneth could continue living as he had. Most healthy people have difficulty imagining a life like Kenneth's, which perhaps seems so desperately limited and uncomfortable that death would be preferable. Yet Kenneth himself had lived that way for 21 years, and his desire to die now was not motivated by any change in his physical health, but by the psychological loss involved in the death of his parents. The court itself described him as "preoccupied with fear over the quality of his life after the death of his father," but did not suggest it would endorse legal immunity for assisting the suicide of *anyone* driven to kill himself by the despair arising from the loss of close family members. "[I]f Kenneth enjoyed sound physical health, but had viewed his life as unbearably miserable because of his mental state", he would have no "right to terminate his life with or without the assistance of others." But given that he was "a competent adult beset by conditions noted above," he had a "right under the common law to withdraw his consent" to continued use of the respirator. In short, the court essentially held that his physical limitations—or perhaps those limitations combined with his psychological fears—gave him the right to bring about his death.

Even if most would find it reasonable to decide that life as a ventilator-dependent quadriplegic is not worth living, is it possible that Kenneth himself would have reached a different view had he been provided more support in adjusting to the loss of his parents? If so, then his decision may have been based upon a treatable transient depression, and for that reason may not have deserved the deference it was given. Our ethical obligation might instead be to provide the necessary support. Yet that course presents practical complications of its own. The missing support may not be entirely psychological. Kenneth's fears about the quality of care he would receive after his father's death necessarily assume an assessment of the facilities that would then be available to him. In this regard the story of Larry McAfee, partially told in *Georgia v. McAfee*, 385 S.E.2d 651 (Ga.1989) is illuminating. McAfee was an avid outdoorsman until a motorcycle accident left him in essentially the same state as Kenneth. He initially made a life for himself as a computer consultant, but later sought judicial permission to die when the quality of his care declined after he was forced to change living arrangements because his insurance settlement was exhausted. Like Kenneth, he prevailed in court, but by then he had found better care and chose to live. Had Kenneth remained alive throughout the appeals process (he died when his father, a week before his own death, gave him a sedative and loosened his tracheostomy tube), the Nevada court might have pursued the matter further. It did note that had Kenneth still been alive, it would have allowed the order he sought "subject only to" Kenneth's consultation with a health care provider or government representative who would have informed him of the care alternatives available to him after his father's death.

McKay's legal analysis follows a catechism traceable back beyond *Perlmutter* to the earlier case of *Saikewicz* (discussed below in Section D.3), which identified four factors that might provide a basis for overriding "the right of an individual to refuse medical treatment." This four-factor discussion has appeared repeatedly in the cases ever since, and we therefore examine all four in turn here, even though they seem to impede rather than assist thoughtful analysis. The four factors are 1) the state's interest in the preservation of life, 2) the duty to prevent suicide, 3) the need to protect innocent third parties, and 4) the need to maintain the ethical integrity of medicine. The first two are hard to distinguish, since the duty to prevent suicide presumably arises from the interest in preserving life. But state courts have traditionally considered them separately.

Perlmutter easily concludes that the state's interest in preserving life fails to justify overriding the patient's decision where, as here, "the condition is terminal, the patient's situation wretched, and the continuation of his life temporary and totally artificial." *McKay* employs similar language, effectively finding the state interest diminished below the necessary threshold whenever a competent patient on life support who is subject to physical and mental suffering decides to die. The California Supreme Court reached much the same result in what would seem a more difficult case. Howard Andrews, while in state prison under a life sentence, became quadriplegic as a result of a fall from a prison wall. He lost sensation in and control over his body below his shoulders, and unlike Kenneth, he was not ventilator-dependent. Depressed over his condition, he refused to eat, and prison physicians sought an order allowing them to insert a gastrojejunostomy tube into his intestines to permit artificial feeding. The court turned them down. It concluded that the state interest in preserving life was inadequate to overrule Howard's choice. The petitioners pointed out that Howard's condition did not impose the same agonies suffered by patients in most earlier cases. His condition, while tragic, was certainly less grim than either Kenneth's or Abe's. The court brushed these points aside. "For self-determination to have any meaning, it cannot be subject to the scrutiny of anyone else's conscience or sensibilities. It is the individual who must live or die with the course of treatment chosen or rejected, not the state. Particularly when the restoration of normal health and vitality is impossible, only the person whose moment-to-moment existence lies in the balance can resolve the difficult and uniquely subjective questions involved." Thor v. Superior Ct., 855 P.2d 375, 384 (Cal.1993). This ringing endorsement of personal autonomy leaves the reader uncertain when, if ever, the interest in preserving life would prevail. The discussion in the case is generally unhelpful on this point.

Indeed, *Thor*'s focus on autonomy may distract one from the important point that the patient here is, after all, a *prisoner*, who as a general matter is unlikely to feel the same sense of choice as the judges, and for whom the state has a correspondingly greater duty. One might ask, for example, whether the prison psychiatrists who diagnosed his depression made any effort to treat it. The court noted but rejected the argument, made by the amici curiae, that "the prison's lack of rehabilitative personnel or facilities, psychological counseling, or necessary physical accommodations of the disability may unduly influence" the prisoner's choice, because, the court said, such limitations may affect persons outside prison as well, and any third party examination of whether they affected Howard's capacity to make a rationale choice "would denigrate the principle of personal autonomy, substituting a species of legal paternalism". This analysis surely leaves the state's interest in preserving life as unlikely ever to prevail. Would the state be allowed to force-feed a suicidal prisoner who was otherwise healthy? *Thor* reserved that question, although the Rhode Island Supreme Court subsequently rejected *Thor*'s application to such a case and authorized the prison director to use all reasonable means, including insertion of a nasogastric feeding tube, to preserve the life of such a prisoner. Laurie v. Senecal, 666 A.2d 806 (R.I.1995).

Judicial discussion of the standard analyses' second factor, prevention of suicide, is usually even more unhelpful. We might define any self-killing as suicide, but usually the term conveys a moral as well as a factual message. One philosophical tradition defines suicide as only wrongful self-killing, just as murder is the wrongful killing of another. The difficult question then lies in deciding when the self-killing is wrongful. The soldier who throws himself on a grenade to protect his fellows would not be described as a suicide under this analysis, but self-killings motivated by self-interest—to escape from difficulties of living—usually would. Killing oneself to avoid pain or unhappiness would usually be regarded as suicide. Perhaps they should not be. Or perhaps we might have a category of justified suicide in which to place some such cases.

But none of the foregoing was addressed by *McKay*, which instead described itself as "attempting to show" that Kenneth had "no intent to take his own life", a remarkable assertion given that it was this very purpose which Kenneth himself believed made his petition necessary. To support its attempt the court offered principally the distinction, discredited in this context, between affirmative acts and allowing death to occur "naturally". Kenneth "sought no affirmative measures to terminate his life; he desired only to eliminate the artificial barriers standing between him and the natural processes

... that would otherwise ensue ...". This is the same odd view of causation examined above in Section A.3 (active vs. passive euthansia). It was also relied on in *Perlmutter*, when that court claimed that Abe Perlmutter's decision was no really suicide because removal of his respirator was not the true cause of his death.

These arguments do not improve with repetition. Neither court would accept this "causation" or "intent" defense of a third party who, pathologically repulsed by the sight of sick people, yanked out Abe's or Kenneth's respirator so as to "let nature to take its course". As the concurring judge in *McKay* observed, Kenneth "did not want to die a 'natural' death; he wanted to die an immediate death." Courts allow Abe and Kenneth to arrange removal of their respirators because the courts believe their desire to end their life is reasonable, not because the courts doubt either their intent to end their life, or the accuracy of their belief that removing the respirator will achieve their purpose. By pretending otherwise, *McKay* misses the opportunity to explore overtly and systematically the necessary elements of what we might call justifiable suicide. Why, for example, does *McKay* suggest that killing oneself from mental dispair alone is not justifiable suicide, while such despair accompanied by a serious but non-terminal illness is? See also *Thor*, which, relying on *McKay*'s motive analysis, concludes, quite remarkably, that Andrews is not committing suicide—and that therefore the prison administrator has no duty to intervene.

The third factor, protection of innocent third parties, is rarely determinative. *Perlmutter* and *McKay* found it inapplicable, since neither patient had minor children or other dependents whose interest the state might seek to protect. Could this factor ever be important enough to override a patient's otherwise effective decision to terminate his care? The case usually cited for that possibility, and relied upon by *Perlmutter,* is Application of the President and Directors of Georgetown College, 331 F.2d 1000 (D.C.Cir.1964). A 25–year old woman lost two-thirds of her blood as a result of a ruptured ulcer. She had a reasonable chance to survive with a blood transfusion, and none without it, but her husband declined to consent because, as a Jehovah's Witness, he believed that transfusions were forbidden by the Bible. He made clear he would not oppose a transfusion ordered by a court, since the responsibility would then not be his. His wife's condition made it difficult to ascertain her views, but they appeared the same as her husband's. The writ was granted within hours, limited to those transfusions necessary to save the patient's life. The opinion noted in a single paragraph that the patient was the mother of a 7 month old child, which gave the state an interest in preserving her life so as to preclude "this most ultimate of voluntary abandonments."

While this provocative language explains the frequent *Georgetown* citation, it is hardly the opinion's main point. To the contrary, the opinion emphasizes that the patient had a reasonable chance to be brought back to health that was put in doubt only because her husband declined to consent to a procedure most would regard as relatively benign. And his opposition was directed more to *authorizing* the transfusion than to the transfusion itself. These facts were sufficient to justify the court's order had the patient been childless: the autonomy principle's relevance is marginalized because the patient herself has not refused the treatment, and there is a stronger basis than in *Perlmutter* upon which to appeal to paternalistic considerations. *Georgetown* is thus best explained by considerations entirely apart from the proposition for which it is most often cited, that a competent patient's decision to decline treatment can be overridden by their duties to third parties. In fact, with one special exception, treated below in Chapter 8, there is little if any authority which clearly relies on the "duty to third party" principle to force treatment on an unwilling patient, even though many cases still list this factor as having potential application. (The exception arises where the patient is pregnant, and the refusal of medical care endangers her unborn child. Even in that case, however, prevailing law is unclear. See Chapter 8.B, *infra*. And there are cases saluting the *Georgetown* principle but finding it inapplicable.)

Nor has the fourth factor (integrity of the medical profession) usually been important. The cases long ago concluded that the ethics of medical practice do not require "all efforts toward life prolongation . . . in all circumstances" (*Satz,* relying on *Saikewicz*). Can the state's interest in maintaining ethical standards in medicine ever justify overriding a competent patient's treatment decision? *McKay* presents the kind of facts most likely to raise this question: where the patient, by virtue of incapacitation, requires the assistance of another person to affirmatively bring about his own death. The state may have an interest in barring doctors from providing such assistance as a cautionary measure intended to avoid any ambiguity, in the minds of both the doctors and others, in their duties to their patients generally. The question was perhaps put most directly in the well-known case of Bouvia v. Superior Ct., 225 Cal.Rptr. 297 (App.1986).

Elizabeth Bouvia suffered since birth from both cerebral palsy and arthritis, and she was quadriplegic by the time she entered the hospital at 28. She had earned a college degree and had married, but her husband had left her. Totally dependent on others for all her needs, including toileting, turning, or sitting upright in bed, she had a tube attached to her chest that automatically injected periodic doses of morphine to relieve her chronic pain. Her parents had cared for her but now felt they no longer could. Dependent on public assistance, she had been unsuccessful in finding a permanent place to live where she could receive the constant care she needed. She thus ended up in the hospital. Although she could eat soft food if spoon fed, hospital staff believed she was not eating enough to maintain her life, and noted an earlier episode at another hospital in which she tried to starve herself to death. Over her objection the hospital inserted a nasogastric tube, and she sought an injunction requiring its removal. She said she would eat as much as she could swallow without nausea and vomiting, and claimed (correctly, it later turned out, although the courts could not then know it) that she could eat enough to stay alive. The trial court found the tube necessary to sustain life and denied the injunction, but on appeal she prevailed, the court holding that she could not be forced to accept artificial feeding even if her life was thereby endangered. In language strongly supportive of patient autonomy and later confirmed by *Thor*, the court held that Bouvia's quality of life was a "significant consideration" justifying the result despite the possibility that with support Bouvia could live 15 or 20 additional years. The decision to terminate treatment was not "a legal question whose soundness is to be resolved by lawyers or judges," but "was [Bouvia's] alone." Although this court also engaged in the usual ritualistic denial that allowing "nature to take its course" could be suicide, it also observed "that a desire to terminate one's life is probably the ultimate exercise of one's right to privacy."

The effect of the court's decision was to require the hospital to treat Bouvia selectively: she was entitled to the pain killers and comfort assistance which she requested, yet the hospital could not ensure that she received the nutrition she required to stay alive. This places hospital personnel in a situation some might find ethically unacceptable: they are compelled to assist a patient in starving herself to death, by keeping her comfortable during the process, which may takes weeks or longer. The situation is more difficult than the case in which a respirator is removed, for there death will typically occur within hours, and the entire process can be carried out by the attending physician acting alone. Implementation of Bouvia's decision, however, necessarily requires the cooperation of wider group of hospital personnel over several weeks or months. It is therefore more likely to require imposing duties on hospital personnel with ethical objections to the patient's decision.

The court noted the state's claimed interest in "maintaining the ethical standards of the medical profession," which included "the right of physicians to effectively render necessary and appropriate medical service and to refuse treatment to an uncooperative and disruptive patient." But it never again refers to these concerns, suggesting that it found them less than persuasive, at least in this case. Yet note that the right of access to abortion does not include a right to require physicians to perform abortions to which they conscientiously object. Nor would it seem that a patient entitled to a lethal dose of morphine would thereby also be entitled to compel a conscientiously objecting physician to administer it. Can Bouvia insist on cooperation from physicians or institutions that have conscientious objections to her request? The court's lack of interest in this question may have resulted from an assumption that the medical personnel's resistance was based on their fear of liability, not on conscientious objection. The concurrence made this assumption explicit. We thus cannot know if they would have reached the same result had such a conscientious objection been plainly made. Of course, the patient faced with such conscientious objection can typically transfer to the care of others more comfortable with her request. That solution may be more difficult to achieve, however, for a patient with an unconventional request that is likely to generate widespread conscientious objection, or one without insurance.

In short, the cases generally support the right of competent patients to refuse or discontinue life-sustaining treatment. Most cases note the same four state interests that might be offered to override the patient's decision, but when the patient is terminally ill, or has physical limitations that severely compromise his quality of life, today courts almost invariably sustain his decision to shorten his life. Less certain is how courts would treat similar claims by sick persons who are not terminally ill, and whose quality of life does not seem intolerably compromised to the court (even if it does to the patient). Such facts would test the broad pro-autonomy language of opinions like *Thor*.

There is another variation of this fact pattern worth noting: the case where recovery is possible, if in a compromised state, but the treatment to achieve it is sufficiently painful or repulsive that some patients may prefer to die. Amputations can present this profile. In the few cases that have arisen, courts usually allow competent patients to die rather than to suffer the trauma of losing a limb. Less often litigated are cases of severe burns, for which treatment requires extremely painful immersions in antibiotic baths, and recovery often comes at the price of disfigurement or loss of function. Dax Cowert believed the pain of treatment was not worth the quality of survival, but he was nonetheless treated over his objection for 14 months. He survived, blind and hearing-impaired, with limited use of hands and arms, and facially scarred. After several difficult years of adjustment, he finally reestablished a life he felt worth living. Married, graduated from law school, and self-supporting, he nonetheless still maintains that the physicians should have heeded his objections and ceased treatment. See *Dax's Case: Essays in Medical Ethics and Human Meaning* (L. Kliever, ed., 1988) and R. Burt, *Taking Care of Strangers* 1–21 (1979). *Bouvia* offers supporting precedent for Cowart's position. Less certain is how a court would handle the nontreatment request of a burn patient with a more favorable prognosis.

4. Assisted Suicide and the Constitutional Claim Generally

Going back at least to *Quinlan*, cases and commentators have often suggested that a patient's right to refuse treatment is part of the constitutionally protected right of privacy. The suggestion is plausible, as the constitutional right of privacy shields similar decisions, such as reproductive choices, from state coercion. But other cases and commentary suggest the constitutional claim may be superfluous, or even a source of difficulty.

Any discussion of the constitutional issues must distinguish among three different kinds of cases. Some cases involve incompetent or unconscious patients, where a constitutional claim to refuse treatment is made by a third party who claims to speak for patient—the situation in Cruzan v. Director, 497 U.S. 261 (1990). While we examine such cases of *surrogate decisionmaking* in subsequent sections, we will deal here with the claim that the decision-making authority accorded the surrogate is constitutionally supported. Second, there are cases in which a currently competent patient declines either to continue a treatment (as in withdrawing a respirator) or to commence a new treatment (such as antibiotic baths for burns). Finally, there are cases in which a competent individual, usually but not necessarily seriously sick, wants to die sooner (or perhaps differently) than he would if he waited for his death to result from untreated illness. Such a person might of course take his own life without need for judicial involvement, but what if he needs another's assistance to end his life, or to end it comfortably? Kenneth McKay needed someone to administer a sedative and loosen his respirator; a terminal cancer patient might seek a physician to administer a lethal dose of morphine. It was a constitutional claim of access to this kind of *assisted suicide* that the Supreme Court rejected in Washington v. Glucksberg, 117 S.Ct. 2258 (1997) and

Vacco v. Quill, 117 S.Ct. 2293 (1997). We discuss these three groups of cases in order.

The first kind of case—where a surrogate acts for an incompetent patient—can arise in two different ways. First, a surrogate might seek merely to follow persuasive evidence of the patient's own views on treatment refusal, definitely expressed at an earlier time when the patient had decisionmaking capacity. Such directions are the patient's, not the surrogate's, and are therefore entitled to whatever deference the Constitution requires we give to the patient's own views. Of course, doubts may be raised about the persuasiveness of the evidence of her views, or about whether the patient would in fact want views she expressed in one context to apply to a situation arising later in another. Ultimately, such doubts may lead us to conclude we do not in fact know the patient's own preference with respect to the decision that *now* must be made. This gives rise to the second version of these cases, in which the issue presented is: how doubt-free must we be before we can act as if we in fact know the patient's own desires? That was essentially the question put in *Cruzan*.

Once Nancy Cruzan was diagnosed as in a permanent vegetative state following her automobile accident, her parents sought to have her disconnected from the tubes that provided her nutrition and water. Missouri would require the doctors to defer to this request only if there was clear and convincing evidence that it was *Nancy*'s wish—a standard the Missouri court held unmet in this case. Affirming, the Supreme Court found nothing in the Constitution required Missouri to apply a more lax evidentiary standard. Even more importantly, the Court made clear that even if there is a Constitutional right to decide on medical treatment (as to which the Court technically reserved judgment), the Due Process Clause does not confer it on "anyone but the patient herself". Legislators might conclude it wise to give decisionmaking authority to close relatives in such cases, but family members have no *constitutional* claim to act for the patient, for "there is no automatic assurance that the view of close family members will necessarily be the same as the patient's would have been had she been confronted with the prospect of her situation while competent."

It may be important to the Court's decision that Nancy had not herself appointed her parents (or anyone else) as her medical decisionmaker, as she might in principle have done by executing a medical power of attorney (discussed below in § D.1) before her accident. Especially under these facts, the Court is surely correct. The claim that the Constitution protects a patient's right to refuse medical treatment must rest on notions of autonomy and personal privacy that by their nature can have no application to a stand-in appointed by the state. If nature deprived Nancy of her ability to decide, the Constitution cannot restore it. Nancy's parents can have no more claim to exercise that constitutional right than they have to exercise her right to vote. See Ira Ellman, *Cruzan v. Harmon and the Dangerous Claim that Others Can Exercise an Incapacitated*

Patient's Right to Die, 29 Jurimetrics J. L. Sci. &
Tech. 389 (1989).

There is another virtue as well in the Court's
decision. Everyone agrees that not every available
medical procedure should forever be provided to an
incompetent patient who left no directions and appointed no agent to decline them. The difficulty lies
in establishing the process for making decisions on
behalf of such patients and the precise boundaries
within which the appointed decisionmaker may act.
There are many factual nuances and difficult policy
choices that must be made in working out such
details, in part because the rules one adopts may
affect physician and hospital behavior in ways that
will impact other patients not before the court.
One's policy judgments may also be affected by the
often rapid changes in medical knowledge and medical technology. Much can be learned from the experiences with the varying solutions chosen by different state courts and legislatures. Invoking the
Constitution to impose a uniform national rule that
can be changed only by decisions of the U.S. Supreme Court, serving in effect as a national board
of bioethics in this field, would almost certainly be
unhelpful.

What then of our second group of cases—those in
which a currently competent patient refuses medical care necessary to keep him alive? Here the
patient acts for himself and the constitutional claim
thus seems more apt. Yet it will typically be superfluous. A constitutional right would protect the
individual from government action only. But

through the battery action the common law long ago established that individuals have a right against unwanted physical intrusions enforceable against private actors like physicians and hospitals. Perhaps that right is not absolute—the common law offers few exceptions—but neither is any possible constitutional right. Any state interest in preserving life and preventing suicide would limit the constitutional right as much as it would shield the battery defendant. If courts typically balance these competing factors in the same way with or without reference to the constitutional doctrine, then nothing is added by it. Some courts have recognized this point. E.g., in *In re* Conroy, 486 A.2d 1209 (N.J.1985), the New Jersey Supreme Court rested entirely on common law principles, choosing to abandon as unnecessary its earlier reliance, in *Quinlan*, on constitutional arguments. And in *Glucksberg*, the Supreme Court noted that the right whose existence it assumed in *Cruzan* was based on "the common law rule that forced medication was a battery."

Where the constitutional claim would have importance is with our third group of cases, involving assisted suicide, because it would go beyond traditional common law principles. The common law does not recognize a right to assist another in dying, even at his request. The victims's consent is no defense to murder. But of course it could be; a state could allow that defense, as Oregon now has, in limited circumstances. Oregon's Death With Dignity Act shields from civil or criminal liability a health care provider who, after certain procedural safeguards are met, provides lethal "medication" to a person expected to die within six months from a terminal disease who has "expressed his or her wish to die" and made a written request for the death potion. Ore.Rev.Stat. § 127.800. Oregon's measure was hotly debated (initially passed in 1995 by the slimmest of margins, it only became effective in 1998 after surviving its own Constitutional challenge, a second public vote, and scrutiny from the federal government as to whether it violated federal drug regulations), but even it would not help someone like Kenneth, the ventilator-dependent quadriplegic whose case (*McKay*) was discussed above. Kenneth was not expected to die within six months, nor could he administer the potion to himself (and nothing in the Act provides immunity to someone who administers it to another). Yet even with these limitations, Oregon's law goes beyond that of any other American jurisdiction.

The stakes were thus high when, in *Glucksberg*, the Court considered a substantive due process challenge to Washington's much more typical law, which made it a felony punishable by up to five years' imprisonment to "knowingly cause or aid another person to attempt suicide". The challenge was brought by physicians who complained that the law kept them from providing their terminally ill patients the assistance they sometimes wanted to end their lives. If the Court had struck down such provisions on their face, the effect would have been to hold that the Constitution compels every state to go further than even Oregon has gone to date.

Framing the question before it narrowly—whether the liberty protected by the Due Process Clause includes "a right to commit suicide which itself includes a right to assistance in doing so"—the Court answered "no". Five justices signed the opinion for the Court, but all nine concurred in the judgment. Agreeing that many of the rights found within protected liberty "sound in personal autonomy", the Court nonetheless rejected the "sweeping conclusion" that all important intimate decisions are so protected, and relied upon the law's historically consistent criminalization of assisted suicide to conclude that it was outside this protected zone. This conclusion rendered inapplicable the cases that protect pregnant women from regulations denying them access to medical assistance necessary for an abortion—a protected liberty *within* that zone. Having thus excluded a more demanding level of scrutiny, the Court considered whether Washington's ban on assisted suicide had the required rational basis. It found four good rationales for the prohibition.

The Court sensibly treated the first, the state's interest in preserving human life, as including the indistinguishable interest in preventing suicide that state court cases so typically list as a second state interest. State court cases like *McKay* and *Thor* (discussed above) find this state interest proportional to the suicidal claimant's quality of life. *Glucksberg* does not bar a state from adopting this sliding view of its own interest. But in this context Washington had not, for its prohibition on assisting suicide (like the statutes of other states) makes no such sliding scale exception. *Glucksberg* reaffirmed that States may assert an interest in preserving human life unaffected by such quality of life judgments. In reaching this result the Court relied in part on concerns that physicians often fail to respond adequately to the pain and depression experienced by the seriously ill, who in turn are then more likely to become suicidal. In short, the Court found Washington's rule a reasonable expression of a policy to favor improvement of the patient's quality of life over termination of it. Washington chose to risk the "error" of keeping alive some whose lives cannot in fact be improved, over the "error" of killing some who would have preferred to live, had they been provided better treatment. The likelihood of each error is an empirical question for which there is probably no good data. In that vacuum it would seem impossible to find Washington's choice irrational.

The three other policies identified by the Court all easily satisfied the test of rationality. The state's interest in protecting the integrity of the medical profession, another familiar member of the usual state-court quartet, had more bite in this context, for § 2.21 of the A.M.A. Code of Ethics itself states that "physician-assisted suicide is fundamentally incompatible with the physician's role as a hearler." A state interest in protecting vulnerable groups from abuse, neglect and mistakes was found relevant; bias or indifference toward the poor, elderly or disabled, when coupled with pressures to reduce expenditures on medical care, might place them at particular risk under a legal regime which drew a less bright line against intentional killing.

Finally, the Court noted Washington's concern that establishing a constitutional right to commit suicide will lead to a broader and even less acceptable practice of euthanasia. Such slippery slope arguments are often unpersuasive, but passing comments by the Court of Appeals in this very case—in the *en banc* opinion which the Court reversed—lent it unintended power. While purporting to draw its constitutional line as protecting only the decision of the patient himself to hasten his own death, the appeals court had also observed that a patient's right could be exercised by "a duly appointed surrogate decisionmaker" and that in some cases a third party, rather than the patient himself, would have to administer the death potion. Justice Souter, who otherwise found the claimed right persuasive, concurred in the Court's judgment, persuaded that the state could reasonably decide that a clear rule against all assisted suicide was necessary to avoid abuse of patients whose desire to die was either absent or the product of neglect or coercion. The right to assisted suicide, he noted, "could not be readily containable by reference to facts about the mind that are matters of difficult judgment, or by gatekeepers who are subject to temptation, noble or not." These are much the same considerations as those explored in section A.3's discussion of the argument some make to distinguish permissible passive euthanasia and impermissible active euthanasia: the former is, by its nature, less susceptible to abuse than the latter.

The same argument is also relied upon by Justice Souter for his concurrence in *Glucksberg*'s companion case, *Vacco v. Quill*, in which the Court rejected plaintiffs' argument that New York (and by implication, all other states) violate the Equal Protection Clause when it distinguishes between aiding another to commit suicide (which is a crime), and refusing medical treatment necessary to sustain one's own life (which is allowed). The Court's brief opinion relies heavily on purported differences in intent and causation to justify the disparate treatment of these two kinds of cases—a weak if classic distinction essentially identical to the arguments used by state courts like *McKay* and *Thor* when they deny that a patient who refuses treatment thereby commits suicide. (Those arguments are criticized in section C.3 above.) This distinction is less persuasive than the slippery slope argument offered in Justice Souter's concurrence.

Glucksberg and *Vacco* do not necessarily end the Constitutional debate, however. As Justice Stevens observed in his concurrence, the Court's rejection of these *facial* challenges to bans on assisted suicide does not necessarily foreclose a successful challenge to such laws *as applied*. For example, such bans can be read to reach the physician who prescribes a strong dose of morphine to ease the suffering of a terminal lung cancer patient, knowing that the dosage will also hasten his death. It is unclear that criminal prosecutions have ever been brought in such cases. But if they were, they might not withstand constitutional scrutiny, given the language not only in Justice Stevens' opinion, but also the similar language in the separate opinion of Justice O'Connor, one of the five justices who signed the opinion for the court.

D. PATIENTS LACKING DECISIONMAKING CAPACITY

1. Patients With Advance Directives

Most states have statutes, often called "Natural Death" acts, that authorize "living wills" in which a person states their wishes about the medical treatment they would want under specified conditions. An alternative to the living will is a medical power of attorney which appoints an agent to make medical decisions if the principal becomes incapable of expressing his preferences. A single document may encompass both approaches: it may appoint another to speak on the maker's behalf, but include specific directions as to the maker's desires. All these documents are called advance directives. After the decision in *Cruzan* Federal law was amended to require hospitals, nursing care facilities, hospices and prepaid health care organizations to disseminate written information to their patients about their rights under local law to accept or refuse care and to formulate advance directives, and to document in the hospital records whether patients have such directives. 42 U.S.C. §§ 1395cc(f)(1) and 1396a(a).

a. *Living Wills*

Early living will statutes often contained restrictive provisions robbing them of much usefulness. For instance, former Calif. Health & Safety Code § 7187(c) limited living wills to authorizing the withdrawal of a procedure that "would serve only to artificially prolong the moment of death ... where ... death is imminent whether or not such procedures are utilized." They were thus inapplicable to patients in persistent vegetative states who might live on, unconscious, for years. (Karen Quinlan died almost ten years after her respirator was removed.) Such hedges, reflecting legislative caution when living wills were first enacted, have now been largely abandoned. Current California law, for instance, allows the living will to authorize withdrawal of "any medical procedure or intervention that, when administered to a [a patient in a coma or terminal condition], will serve only to prolong the process of dying or an irreversible coma or persistent vegetative state." Calif. Health & Safety Code § 7186. Living wills nonetheless continue to be of limited value. If they permit only the withdrawal of life-sustaining treatment, they cannot provide a basis for affirmative acts such as the humane administration of morphine to the terminally ill cancer patient in great pain. They also do not address situations, increasingly common, of patients in a severely debilitated and mentally compromised state who may be suffering greatly, but who are nevertheless not technically terminal or in a permanent vegetative state. Several examples can be found in the cases discussed below.

Living wills are also criticized by those who believe that even if autonomy principles justify great deference to a patient's contemporaneous decisions, these principles offer less support to advance directives in which individuals attempt to anticipate what they will wish done in the future under circumstances they have never directly experienced. Are the interests and values of a competent person even still relevant when they lose competency? If not, is it appropriate to leave the fate of the current person in the hands of their prior self? See John Robertson, *Second Thoughts About Living Wills*, 21 Hastings Center Rep., Nov.–Dec. 1991. The more specific the living will attempts to be in describing the alternative possible future circumstances, and the desired treatment in each, the greater is the likelihood that the present self is ignorant of facts that would be important to the future self who will be bound by these directions. Yet directives that leave only general guidelines or principles of decision may leave the future self at the mercy of whoever has responsibility for construing them, which may be medical personnel unknown to the present self. One survey by Joan Teno and Joanne Lynn found that of 4,804 terminally ill patients, only 688 had any advance directive, and only 22 of these 688 contained instructions explicit enough to guide medical care. *Living Wills Are Rarely of Aid, a Study Says*, New York Times, 4/8/97, at A9.

b. Durable Powers of Attorney

For most people a durable power of attorney conferring medical decisionmaking authority on a family member or friend chosen by the principal is a better choice than a living will. (A power of attorney is "durable" when it provides expressly that the agent's authority continues even when the principal becomes incompetent; without such language, the agent's authority lapses at that point.) Some states provide specially for "medical" powers of attorney, distinguishing them from more general durable powers of attorney provided for in the law of every state, and most typically used to confer authority over the principal's financial affairs. Even if state law does not explicitly recognize such medical powers of attorney, the broad language usually contained in the general statutes is reasonably interpreted to permit appointment of an agent with medical decisionmaking authority, as some state courts have held. One way or another, such an appointment of a proxy medical decisionmaker is allowed in the majority of states, and avoids many of the difficulties present with living wills. The principal relies on the judgment of a person close to her who is familiar with the principal's values, rather than on explicit directions which may fail to anticipate all the circumstances.

State statutes on medical powers of attorney, as well as those authorizing living wills, typically limit their scope to patients who are terminally ill, permanently comatose, or in a persistent vegetative state. In addition, both kinds of statutes often limit or even disallow the refusal of nutrition and hydration, as contrasted with other medical treatment. Living will statutes also often suspend or otherwise limit their application to patients who are pregnant.

2. Once–Competent Patients Without Advance Directives

Most patients do not have formal advance directives, and those who do often do not address the precise situation at hand. How do we then make medical care decisions for them? Should we rely on any available evidence of their likely preference, or instead on what is generally considered to be best for them? Courts are torn between these two conflicting impulses. On one hand, they are anxious, if at all possible, to ground a decision to withdraw treatment on the patient's own choice—to rely on the autonomy principle. On the other hand, serious doubts exist about our ability to discern an intent that was never formally expressed, on the basis of statements in informal conversations conducted in very different circumstances, especially where the purported intent is contrary to what many patients would want.

This tension is reflected in the two competing legal rules that courts apply in making decisions for incapacitated patients. The objective "best interests" test asks which course of action is in the patient's best interests. The alternative favored by many courts is the "substituted judgment" rule, under which the court attempts to make the same decision it believes the patient would have made, if the patient were not incapacitated. In applying a substituted judgment approach to a patient who left no advance directive but once had decisionmaking capacity, the court must examine whatever evidence is available about the patient's values and preferences concerning death and dying issues.

New Jersey has been a leading proponent of the substituted judgment approach, but it also allows reliance on objective assessments in cases where the patient's views are not accessible. The evolution of the New Jersey rule began in *Quinlan,* in which the New Jersey supreme court found that statements Karen had once made in casual conversations, about heroic measures for terminally ill patients, were "remote and impersonal" and therefore "lacked significant probative weight." Must the court following a substituted judgment approach then conclude that life must be maintained because there is no basis in the patient's own views to terminate support, or shall it instead abandon substituted judgment for an objective best interests standard? As the New Jersey rule ultimately evolved, courts may consider evidence of the patient's probable intentions that is less persuasive than instructions in a formal advance directive, by giving it proportionately less weight. This modulated approach was developed in the companion cases of In re Jobes, 529 A.2d 434 (N.J.1987) and In re Peter, 529 A.2d 419 (N.J.1987).

Peter involved a 65 year old nursing home patient in an irreversible coma, a state in which she could live "indefinitely." The question was whether to

remove a nasogastric tube that sustained her with
essential nutrients and fluids. The court held it
could be removed if there was "clear and convincing
evidence" she would have wanted it removed—the
same test that Missouri had applied in *Cruzan*, and
which the Supreme Court held constitutionally permissible. But in *Peter*, unlike *Cruzan*, the court
found the test was met. Before she lost decisionmaking capacity Peter had not only made her intentions clear, she had executed a a medical power of
attorney appointing a friend who now directed the
tube's removal. The court held that the tube could
be removed without regard to the impact on the
patient's life expectancy and without engaging in
any objective balancing of the treatment's burdens
and benefits. The patient's own views had been
demonstrated with sufficient certainty to provide a
basis for proceeding without need for those inquiries.

In *Jobes*, by contrast, the evidentiary test was not
met. The medical facts were similar: a 31 year old
woman, in a coma following an automobile accident,
was sustained by a j-tube inserted in her abdomen
that provided her with essential nutrients and made
it possible for her to continue indefinitely. She had
already been in a coma for seven years at the time
of the court's decision. The question was whether
the j-tube could be withdrawn, as her husband had
requested. Unlike Peters, Nancy Jobes had left no
clear evidence of her desires, and the court concluded that, despite his efforts to show that Nancy
would have agreed, the husband was expressing his

views as to her interests rather than her own. But it nonetheless held that the doctors could follow his instructions. In the absence of the patient's own directions, "family members are best suited to make substituted judgments for incompetent patients not only because of their peculiar grasp of the patient's approach to life, but also because of their special bonds with him or her. Our common human experience informs us that family members are generally most concerned with the welfare of the patient." *Id.* at 445. New Jersey's willingness to rely on the judgment of family members when the patient herself has left no clear directions distinguishes it from the Missouri rule sustained in *Cruzan*. Recall the Supreme Court there concluded that Missouri's reluctance to rely on the family had a rational basis. Of course, New Jersey's different policy choice is rational as well.

Indeed, the conflicting pressures can be seen in the *Jobes* opinion itself. The court, desirous to portray the decision as Nancy's rather than its own, explains its reliance upon her family as grounded on their special ability to determine what she would have wanted. But because the court also concluded that no one could actually say with confidence what Nancy Jobes would have wanted, it also assures itself that Nancy has a "warm, loving" family who will be "most concerned" with her welfare in making the decision. Because the difficulty here—do we or don't we know what she wanted?—is obvious to the court as well, it restricts the family's right to request withdrawal of care to cases in which the patient is in an irreversible coma. Indeed, the court specifies that for hospitalized patients, a hospital prognosis committee must confirm the medical judgment that the patient is in an irreversible coma, and for nonhospitalized patients like Jobes herself (she was in a nursing home), two independent physicians must confirm the prognosis. In addition, doctors who have doubts about the instructions given them by family members can seek appointment of a guardian to review their decision. The decisionmaking authority of family members in cases like *Jobes* is thus considerably circumscribed, as compared to the friend who held the patient's power of attorney in *Peter*. In effect, *Jobes* allows family members to withdraw life sustaining measures only in those cases—irreversible coma—where the court would probably reach the same result applying a more objective best interests standard.

What then do we do in cases where the patient is not in a coma, so that *Jobes* does not apply, but has not left clear instructions, so that *Peter* does not apply? In *Peter* the court also reviewed and largely reaffirmed an earlier decision, In re Conroy, 486 A.2d 1209 (N.J.1985), which dealt with such a case. Claire Conroy was an elderly nursing home patient; she was not in a coma, but suffered from severe, permanent, mental and physical impairments. She had left no clear instructions. Her life expectancy was less than a year regardless of what was done for her. As explained later in *Peter,* Conroy's short life expectancy was very important. Where such a patient has a life expectancy of more than a year if treatment is provided, then it cannot be withheld. Even when life expectancy is less than a year, the court imposes important conditions on the family authority to authorize the withholding or withdrawal of life sustaining treatment. The court divides such cases into two groups, depending upon one's knowledge of the patient's probable preferences.

Where one has some "trustworthy" evidence that the patient would have refused further treatment (but that evidence falls short of meeting *Peter*'s "clear and convincing" test, since if it did *Peter* would allow ending treatment without further inquiry), one may still withdraw the treatment if the burdens of the patient's continued life with treatment "markedly outweigh" the benefits the patient may derive from that life. In evaluating whether evidence of the patient's preferences is sufficiently trustworthy, the *Conroy* court found that it had erred in *Quinlan* in disregarding Karen's statements to friends; such evidence was certainly "relevant." Nonetheless, the probative value of such evidence "may vary depending upon the remoteness, consistency, and thoughtfulness of the prior statements or actions and the maturity of the person" at the time, as well as upon the statements' "specificity." Where one does not have trustworthy evidence of the patient's preference, it is not enough that the pain and suffering of continued life "markedly outweigh" the benefits. Before withdrawal of treatment can be allowed for such a patient, one must also find that the patient will

suffer so much pain that prolonging his life "would
be inhumane."

The New Jersey supreme court has addressed
these questions more comprehensively than any
other American court, and its opinions are de-
servedly influential. It is therefore important to
appreciate their emphasis on the autonomy principle as the principle basis upon which care may be
withdrawn. The New Jersey trio do not make it
easy to withdraw care from a patient who has never
expressed clear views in support of that course. If
such a patient is not in an irreversible coma, and
might live for more than a year with full support,
treatment must continue. Even if the noncomatose
patient's life expectancy is less than a year, treatment cannot be terminated in the absence of "inhumane" levels of pain, unless we have trustworthy
evidence that the patient would want care withdrawn. While New Jersey has thus accepted the
possibility of terminating life sustaining care on the
basis of objective determinations of the patient's
best interests rather than the patient's own judgments, it has carefully limited that possibility. A
concurring judge felt the limitations were too great
because the court's emphasis on pain avoidance as
the objective measure of the patient's best interests
"effectively negates other ... considerations....
[S]ome people abhor dependence on others as much,
or more, than they fear pain." The *Conroy* majority's emphasis on pain is nonetheless consistent with
the cautions expressed in Justice Stevens' and
O'Connor's *Glucksberg* opinions.

Other courts depart in both directions from this New Jersey approach. New York, like Missouri in *Cruzan*, allows withdrawal of life sustaining care only on the patient's own authorization, leaving little if any room for employment of more objective factors in cases in which the patient's views are inaccessible. New York's views are set out in In re Mary O'Connor, 534 N.Y.S.2d 886 (N.Y.1988), which involved a 77 year-old woman who had been institutionalized continuously since suffering a stroke three years earlier. She had a major heart attack the year before the stroke. The doctors agreed that she had suffered significant brain damage rendering her permanently incapable of participating in her medical care decisions, but she was not comatose. She could respond to simple commands ("turn over"), and was at times able to sit up in a chair. Her case came to court because she had lost her gag reflex, making it impossible for her to swallow food. Her doctors wanted to insert a nasogastric tube but her two daughters opposed it. They understood that without it she would die of either thirst or starvation. It was uncertain whether Mary O'Connor had the capacity to experience suffering from thirst or starvation, but a physician testified that one could give O'Connor pain killers in any event.

The New York Court of Appeals rejected the daughters' claim, under a standard allowing care to be terminated only when "it was established by clear and convincing evidence that the patient would have so directed if he were competent and

able to communicate." Mary O'Connor had left no
clear instructions on such matters when competent;
the daughters could only report on a few casual
conversations in which she suggested that she
would not want to be sustained artificially. But she
had never discussed the withdrawal of food and
water, nor said whether she would want care withdrawn even "if that would produce a painful
death." This kind of evidence fell well short of the
New York standard. Mary O'Connor's statements
"that nature should be permitted to take its
course" might well have been no more than an
"immediate reaction" to seeing another's prolonged
death, and her saying she would not want to be "a
burden" to anyone is the kind of statement that
older people "invariably make"; "few nursing home
patients would ever receive life sustaining medical
treatment" if such statements were sufficient.

The court of appeals emphasized that "[T]he
right to decline treatment is personal"; that "the
inquiry in New York is limited to ascertaining and
then effectuating the patient's expressed wishes";
and that "the clear and convincing evidence standard requires proof . . . that the patient held a firm
and settled commitment to the termination of life
supports under the circumstances like those presented." These standards were met in the earlier
case of Brother Fox (decided as a companion to
Matter of Storar, 438 N.Y.S.2d 266 (N.Y.1981)), but
not here. Brother Fox was a member of a religious
order "who had conscientiously discussed his moral
and personal views concerning the use of a respira-

tor on persons in a vegetative state." *O'Connor* does not explicitly provide, as does New Jersey, for more relaxed standards where the patient is permanently comatose or likely to die within the year. Because Mary O'Connor was neither, the question was not unavoidably put, but the *O'Connor* opinion offers little basis to predict flexibility on the question—as noted by the dissenters. The New Jersey opinions themselves are ignored by the New York majority.

One thing that should be clear is that no special significance is reasonably attached to the fact that *O'Connor* involved withdrawal of the nasogastric tube providing fluids or nutrition, rather than of medication or respiratory support. Recall, for example, that *Jobes* involved the removal of a j-tube that provided nourishment directly to the patient's small intestine, a point of which the court took no special note. Courts would surely react differently to a plan to deny an immobilized hospital patient food or water he was capable of taking orally. Most courts distinguish between providing food or water, and providing "nutrition" and "hydration" artificially. The first is part of basic humane care that can never be denied; the second is a form of medical treatment that can be withheld or withdrawn on the same basis as any other treatment. This majority approach is consistent with Opinion 2.18 of the AMA Council, which allows the discontinuance of "all means of life-prolonging treatment" for a patient whose coma is "beyond doubt irreversible," and which defines "life prolonging medical treatment" as including "artificially or technologically supplied respiration, nutrition, or hydration."

Any lingering doubt about the appropriateness of treating nasogastric tubes and the like as one treats medication rather than as one treats the provision of food should be set to rest by the analogy to respiration. Food and water are hardly more basic to human life than air. Yet while it is obvious that no court or ethicist would ever consider confining a patient in an airtight room to die of suffocation, it has become routine to withdraw respirators from patients unable to breathe on their own. Food, water, and air are not themselves medical treatments, but the method of delivering them is when a patient is unable to breathe or ingest on his own. One can see this distinction operating in the case of Elizabeth Bouvia, discussed above: essential to her final vindication was her willingness to eat as much as she comfortably could. Once assured of that, the court was willing to require the hospital to follow her wishes and cease providing nutrition and hydration technologically. Elizabeth Bouvia could not compel the hospital to sit by while she starved herself to death, if she were capable of eating on her own, but she could reject the "medical treatment" of a nasogastric tube. *O'Connor* thus applies to any medical treatment, and is not explained by the fact that it involved a feeding tube. Its distinctiveness is instead in the demanding test it applies to deciding whether to withdraw medical care: there must be good evidence that the patient himself favors that course.

Brophy v. New England Sinai Hosp., 497 N.E.2d 626 (Mass.1986) also deviates from the New Jersey approach, but in the opposite direction than New York. Paul Brophy, permanently comatose and unable to swallow, could be sustained for several more years by a G-tube that supplied hydration and nutrients directly to his digestive system. His family wanted the G-tube discontinued, but the hospital refused. He had no living will nor medical power of attorney; but according to his family had said at the hospital, after the rupture of his aneurysm, "If I can't sit up to kiss one of my beautiful daughters, I may as well be six feet under." (There were some other comments more remote in time and context.) New Jersey would have honored the family's facts under *Jobes*, given Brophy's comatose state. But Massachusetts did not limit its holding to comatose patients, and hardly even asked whether it had adequate evidence of the patient's desires. It instead treated the family's instructions as if they were the patient's own, honoring their request as a "substituted judgment."

The family's decision may well have been both sensible and sensitive to Paul Brophy's general approach to life, but the decision was theirs, not Paul Brophy's; probably based as much on what they felt was good for him as on what they could tell he would have wanted. Massachusetts' version of the substituted judgment rule is thus less carefully limited than New Jersey's to cases presenting hard evidence of what the patient would want, even though both courts use the same term. The ap-

proach of the *Brophy* majority led a dissenting judge
to observe that it is "an error of great magnitude to
conflate a substituted judgment with an actual judgment. Such a mistake is ... a blow against individual autonomy.... It is paternalism masquerading
as the mere ratification of autonomous choice."
O'Connor explicitly rejected *Brophy* with the observation that "[N]o person or court should substitute
its judgment as to what would be an acceptable
quality of life for another." 534 N.Y.S.2d at 892.

O'Connor may seem too cautious to many, but
cases do occasionally arise to give one pause. In a
subsequent case, a New York trial judge arguably
went beyond *O'Connor* in issuing an order allowing
the removal of a feeding tube from an 86 year-old
stroke victim who had been in a coma for four and a
half months, and whom doctors had concluded was
in a permanent vegetative state, but whose own
views had not been clearly established. Over the
weekend following the issuance of the order, but
before the doctors acted, the woman awoke. Her
physician was called to her bedside, found her alert,
and proceeded to describe her legal case to her. She
indicated she understood, and the physician then
asked her what she wanted done. "She replied
'These are difficult decisions' and lapsed back into
sleep." The judge then withdrew his order. N.Y.
Times, April 15, 1989, at pg. A15.

Did this trial judge really go beyond the *O'Connor*
standard? While the language of both *Brophy* and
O'Connor are quite different than New Jersey's, as
well as from each other, on the facts before them

both courts would in fact have reached the same result as New Jersey. Perhaps New York and Massachusetts use sweeping language in their opinions only because neither court has yet been forced to face more difficult cases challenging the general approach each seems to adopt. Some insight into this question is provided by examining the cases of patients who have never had decisionmaking capacity, such as the severely retarded. Massachusetts and New York have each decided such a case.

3. Never–Competent Patients

It would not seem possible to employ a true substituted judgment approach with patients who have never possessed decisionmaking capacity. How can one ask what the patient would have wanted, when by definition the patient has never had the capacity to form a view entitled to such deference? It would therefore seem that the only basis for withdrawing life-sustaining treatment in such cases would be an objective judgment that continuation of the treatment would not be in the patient's interests. A state like New York that is resistant to withholding life-sustaining treatment on any basis other than the patient's own views will thus be inclined to always treat the never-competent patient. Consider, for example, *In re Storar*, 438 N.Y.S.2d 266 (N.Y.1981).

John Storar was 52 years old at the time of this case, but his mental age was 18 months. He had been institutionalized since he was five years old. His mother, now 77, visited him "almost daily."

Storar had bladder cancer, which the doctors initially treated with radiation therapy after obtaining his mother's consent. Remission was achieved, but 9 months later the cancer recurred and was diagnosed as terminal. Thereafter the doctors sought to give Storar blood transfusions. He required two units every eight to fifteen days to replace blood losses. The transfusions would not cure his cancer, but without them he had insufficient oxygen in his blood stream, requiring his heart to work harder and causing general lethargy. "After the transfusions he had more energy. He was able to resume most of his usual activities—feeding himself, showering, taking walks, running—including some mischievous ones, such as stealing cigarette butts and attempting to eat them."

Storar would die in three to six months from the cancer, no matter what was done. He might die sooner without the blood transfusions. He had no comprehension of the purpose of the treatment and occasionally resisted it, but in this case the doctors persisted: Storar was given sedatives before the transfusions to eliminate his apprehension. Nonetheless, his mother opposed the treatment. As summarized by the court, her view was rather straightforward: John obviously disliked the transfusions and tried to avoid them, and he should therefore be left alone. The doctors sought a court order to authorize the transfusions. The trial court agreed with Storar's mother, but the New York Court of Appeals reversed.

The Court of Appeals' reasoning was not elaborate. Dismissing any possibility of looking to John Storar's wishes as a guide, it treated the case as one involving an infant whose parents have decided against treatment. While courts cannot second guess the decisions of parents choosing among reasonable alternative treatments, "they may not deny a child all treatment for a condition which threatens his life. The case of a child who may bleed to death because of the parents' refusal to authorize a blood transfusion is a classic example." Storar had terminal cancer, but he also had a blood loss which threatened to end his life sooner, and which was treatable "without excessive pain," even though, due to his incapacity, he did not like the treatment.

Does *Storar* suggests that New York will require treatment of incompetents in all cases? Perhaps not. The *Storar* opinion treats as relevant both the transfusion's effect of increased health and the relatively benign nature of its administration, suggesting the court actually sought to decide for itself where the patient's interests lay. Certainly the result in *Storar* is a plausible outcome of such an objective best interests evaluation. It seems likely New Jersey would reach the same result on the *Storar* facts. Although it has reserved the question of how to deal with the patient who has never been competent, the New Jersey standard for once-competent patients who left no instructions would require treatment: Although John Storar's life expectancy was less than a year, beneficial treatment was available, and he clearly was not suffering so much pain that continuing treatment would be "inhumane." The pain he did suffer seemed controllable with narcotics.

One may contrast *Storer* with Superintendent of Belchertown State School v. Saikewicz, 370 N.E.2d 417 (Mass.1977), where the court contrived to apply the substituted judgment standard to a never-competent patient, authorizing withdrawal of treatment in a straight-faced reliance upon the unacknowledged fiction that it knew the patient's views.

Joseph Saikewicz had been severely retarded since birth. When the case arose he was 67 years old with a mental age of two years and eight months. He had never learned to talk and communicated entirely through physical gestures and grunts. He had lived at the Belchertown State School since 1928, and effectively had no family. Saikewicz had leukemia, for which chemotherapy was the only possible treatment. About half of all patients in his condition achieved a remission of their symptoms with chemotherapy, although many then had recurrence after some months. Without chemotherapy Saikewicz was likely to live only a couple of months at best, and perhaps only a few weeks. Chemotherapy of course often has serious side effects including, in cases like this, nausea, bladder irritation, numbness, tingling of the extremities, and loss of hair. Some side effects can be controlled by other drugs. It was uncontested that "most people in Saikewicz's position elect to suffer the side effects of chemotherapy rather than to allow their leukemia to run its natural course." Nonetheless, a guardian ad litem, appointed on the petition of the School, recommended that Saikewicz not be treated, and this recommendation was accepted by the trial judge. The Massachusetts supreme judicial court affirmed.

The opinion explaining this result is an elaborate exercise in self-deception. Even though Joseph Saikewicz never had the capacity to form any desire, understanding, or opinion on the question of his treatment, the court insisted that "the effort to bring the substituted judgment into step with the values and desires of the affected individual must not, and need not, be abandoned." How can that be done? In what may be one of the most nonsensical statements any court has ever made, the *Saikewicz* majority explained that "the decision . . . should be that which would be made by the incompetent person, if that person were competent, but taking into account the present and future incompetency of the individual. . . ." When urged to follow this Massachusetts approach a few years later, New York, in *Storar*, concluded that to ask what the incompetent would have chosen, if competent, "would be similar to asking whether if it snowed all summer would it then be winter?."

How could Massachusetts implement such an incoherent standard? The opinion is not entirely consistent, but in portions it appears to treat the recommendation of the guardian ad litem as if it were the considered judgment of a competent patient. This portion of the *Saikewicz* opinion discusses the importance of vindicating the patient's right of autonomy, and of honoring his constitutional right to decline treatment. Indeed, at one point the court frames the question before it as reconciling the state's interest in prolonging life with "the interest of an individual to reject the traumatic cost of that prolongation," as if Saikewicz himself had determined he was unwilling to endure the side effects of chemotherapy. In these parts of the opinion the court seems to endow the guardian with the mythical persona of the hypothetically competent Joseph Saikewicz. Yet it is clear that however she might try to interpret the court's standard, the guardian's decision will—at best—reflect the result the guardian imagines she would want for herself were she to be in Saikewicz' situation. That is, in effect, a best interest standard. The problem in *Saikewicz* is not the court's *de facto* use of a best interest standard—what other standard could be used?—but its pretense that it was instead deciding by substituted judgment. That pretense is a problem because it allows the court to shed responsibility for the decision by pretending it is applying the patient's judgment—as expressed by the guardian— rather than its own. Yet the guardian's judgment is not entitled to the special deference arising from the autonomy principle, for it is a judgment that one person has made about another, not a judgment that the patient has made about himself.

Some portions of the *Saikewicz* opinion seem to recognize this reality. These portions try to justify the guardian's recommendation as being in Saikewicz's interest. But the case for justification was difficult given the court's concession that most competent people in Saikewicz's position would choose to be treated. The court therefore had to identify some significant factor weighing against treatment that was present here but not present generally. It identified two possibilities: Saikewicz's inability to cooperate with treatment, and "the quality of life possible for him even if treatment does bring about remission." The court "firmly rejected" the proposition that Saikewicz, on account of his mental retardation, should be allowed to die when others would be treated, because the quality of a retarded person's life is too low. "[T]he chance of a longer life carries the same weight for Saikewicz as for any other person, the value of life under the law having no relation to intelligence. . . . " That left, as the only possible factor peculiar to Saikewicz's case, the impact of chemotherapy on him and his ability to cooperate in the treatment.

Because Saikewicz would have no comprehension of the reasons for "the severe disruption" of his life and routine which chemotherapy would require, the court argued that he "would experience fear without the understanding from which other patients draw strength," and that this problem would be compounded by the "possibility" that "such a naturally uncooperative patient would have to be physically restrained to allow the slow intravenous administration of drugs." Yet Saikewicz's incomprehension could not alone justify denying him treatment, or we would never treat babies—nor would New York have treated Storar. The real issue seemed to be that *Saikewicz*, perhaps on account of his incomprehension, would have to be restrained. Richard Burt, in an insightful commentary in Taking Care of Strangers (1979), concluded that in the trial court at least, the problems of administering the treatment were crucial to the decision against it. The trial transcript suggests that the judge was on the verge of ordering treatment when the attending physicians, present at the hearing, voiced their concern about being required to enter into a struggle with Saikewicz: "When you approach him in the hospital he flails at you and there is no way of communicating with him and he is quite strong; so he will have to be restrained." Yet there was never any effort to determine whether Saikewicz's cooperation could somehow be obtained, perhaps with the aid of institutional staff familiar to him, or by use of sedatives—the kind of tactic employed the doctors in *Storar*. Burt concludes that "this omission reflected everyone's unwillingness to enter into sustained interaction with Joseph Saikewicz, everyone's wish to absent themselves from any transaction with him."

One cannot know for certain why the court did not examine the possibilities for administering treatment to him more carefully before deciding to let him die. But it does appear that this omission was made easier by the court's pretense that it was applying Saikewicz' own decision rather than making a decision for him. The court's concluding paragraph effectively displays its self-deception. "Finding no state interest sufficient to counterbalance a patient's decision to decline life-prolonging medical treatment in the circumstances of this case, we conclude that the patient's right to privacy and self-determination is entitled to enforcement." One can only marvel at the court's ability to transform a case presenting the question of whether others should decide to end Saikewicz's life, into one in which the question is whether the court can keep him from making that choice.

The patient who has never had decisionmaking capacity presents perhaps the hardest case, because we cannot rely at all on the autonomy principle. Courts like *Saikewicz* that pretend to do so do not help resolve the difficult but unavoidable question of deciding when there are objective indicators of the patient's interests that justify stopping treatment.

4. The Seriously Ill Child, Including the Newborn

a. The General Framework of Child Protective Laws

Legally, the child's situation is different from that of the incapacitated adult. No person has legal authority to speak for another adult unless specifically appointed to do so by either that adult himself, in a power of attorney, or by a court, through appointment as the patient's guardian or conservator. But in the case of a child, the parents acquire that authority at birth, and retain it unless and until a court orders otherwise. So when the patient is a child, the question is whether a particular parental decision on medical treatment should be overruled by the court. Although the child possesses no autonomous rights himself, the parent normally speaks for the child, and usually the law treats parental decisions on their child's medical care as dispositive, as if they were the expressed view of a competent adult patient about his own care. Is this level of deference to parental decisions appropriate? That is basically the question presented by the cases addressed here.

The authority to overrule the parental decision arises from state laws designed to protect children from neglectful or abusive parents. Once the threshold finding of abuse or neglect is made, as defined and required under these state laws, courts typically have fairly wide discretion in designing a remedy, which can include the temporary or even permanent removal of the child from the parents' home. Most cases of medical neglect, however, involve one very focused remedy: the authorization of a particular medical procedure or course of treatment, overriding parental objections. To effect such a remedy the court may appoint a temporary guardian to make medical care decisions for the child, either generally or in connection with a particular illness, or the court may simply overrule a single parental decision, and not otherwise intrude. For example, the court might authorize a blood transfusion necessary to preserve the life of a child whose parents will not consent because of their religious scruples.

Abuse and neglect laws are usually triggered by parental decisions to decline necessary medical care, but in theory the imposition of useless or harmful medical care could also be reviewed. Both possibilities are presented simultaneously in cases involving parents who seek to substitute unorthodox procedures for standard medical practice. The New York Court of Appeals faced such a case in In re Hofbauer, 419 N.Y.S.2d 936 (N.Y.1979) involving a seven-year-old child with Hodgkin's disease, a form of cancer. Joey's parents had rejected the advice of their attending physician to immediately commence conventional treatment, including radiation and possibly chemotherapy, but instead brought him to a clinic in Jamaica employing "nutritional or metabolic therapy, including injections of laetrile." On their return a neglect petition was filed. Pending its resolution, the parents were permitted to continue this unconventional therapy under the supervision of a New York physician who favored it. At the hearing the state presented other physicians who testified that the nutritional therapy was ineffective, that Joey's disease had progressed while under it, that conventional therapy offered a prospect of cure, and that if left untreated Hodgkin's disease is almost always fatal. The parents' medical witnesses claimed that Joey had responded well to the nutritional therapy, and the doctor in charge of managing it stated that he "never ruled out the possibility of conventional treatment if the boy's condition appeared to be deteriorating beyond control."

The parents' ability to present supportive medical testimony for their unconventional choice of therapy proved virtually dispositive as the New York court analyzed the matter. Relying heavily on the basic proposition that "great deference" must be paid to the parent's choice of treatment and of physician, the court concluded that, so long as Joey's treatment was supervised by a physician duly licensed in the state of New York, and thus recognized by the state "as capable of exercising acceptable clinical judgment," and so long as the treatment in question "has not been totally rejected by all responsible medical authority," the neglect petition could not succeed. In reaching this result the court found "significant" the testimony of Joey's father that he would accept conventional therapy if so advised by the physician who was managing the nutritional therapy.

New York's approach in *Hofbauer,* while not without any support, is certainly more deferential to parental authority than are many other cases. It contrasts with the Massachusetts decision in the strikingly similar case of Chad Green, which came before the court twice. Custody of a Minor, 379 N.E.2d 1053 (Mass.1978); 393 N.E.2d 836 (Mass. 1979). Chad's leukemia had responded to chemotherapy but recurred when the parents, unbeknownst to the attending physician and contrary to his specific instructions, discontinued his medication. Treatment was resumed under court order and again proved effective, but the parents sought permission from the court to supplement the chemotherapy with "metabolic therapy" consisting of laetrile, vitamins, enzyme enemas and folic acid. Here also the parents produced some medical evidence in support of their position, but the state's physicians were adamantly opposed, insisting, *inter alia,* that the laetrile would actually harm the child. The Massachusetts courts denied the parents' request. They then fled with Chad to Mexico, where he received laetrile but no chemotherapy.

Certainly some people would argue that the adult cancer patient with decisionmaking capacity should have the right to refuse conventional therapy in favor of laetrile, "nutritional therapy," or "metabolic therapy," even where medical authorities are virtually unanimous in their condemnation of such alternative treatments. The adult's right to pursue such unorthodox treatment would surely be based on the autonomy principle. But while the autonomy principle applies to treatment decisions made by parents for themselves, it does not apply to decisions made for their children. Such parental authority is instead one part of a larger tradition of parental prerogatives. Parents vary enormously in their values, their educational choices, their religious views, and their child-rearing philosophies; the general American approach is to acknowledge and protect such diversity, within broad limits. We do this in part because we believe that child-rearing choices are part of a private sphere in which personal values must be protected. But we also impose limits on parental choices that go beyond the limits we place on one's right to make decisions for oneself, because the child is not the parent, but another person whose welfare is an important competing concern.

This tension between respect for parental prerogative and concern for child welfare is reflected in American constitutional law, which invests parental rights with constitutional status, but which also routinely allows the state to override parental claims to require that children attend school, receive required inoculations, and be removed from the custody of parents who abuse them. The cases of Joey Hofbauer and Chad Green required the respective courts to balance these competing claims of parental prerogative and child protection. Clearly, courts will not always strike this balance in the same way as one another. Such balancing can also be heavily affected by how facts are presented. In the end, both Joey Hofbauer and Chad Green died as a result of their parent's refusal to provide them with conventional medical treatment. Yet even though these outcomes seem to vindicate Massachusetts' views, if not its ability to implement them, we can still be sympathetic with the dilemma faced by the New York courts in Joey's case. After all, they did have testimony from a licensed physician defending the parents' decision. To override it would have required them to become intimately involved in a choice which is not normally theirs, a choice between competing treatments each recommended by a properly licensed physician. One might well argue, in fact, that the problem in that case lay not with the analysis of the Court of Appeals, but with the failure of the trial attorneys for the state to present persuasive evidence of the scientific con-

demnation of the laetrile treatment the parents
sought.

Yet the more we try to bring such medical evidence into the courts, the more we are relying on
judges to weigh competing medical claims involving
matters generally beyond their competence. It is
just this problem of how to handle medical uncertainty that pervades many of the difficult newborn
cases. In the case of newborns, however, the drama
of these cases resulted in so much attention that
the federal government inserted itself into the child
protective process, first with regulatory action, and
eventually through Congressional action.

b. The Special Case of the Newborn

One of the major advances of modern medicine is
its vastly improved ability to treat the severely ill
newborn. The most common source of newborn
difficulties is premature birth, but newborn intensive care units at major hospitals now routinely
succeed in ensuring the survival of infants born as
early as 26 weeks gestational age. Surgical procedures have been developed to correct various specific newborn defects, such as spina bifida and hydrocephalus. But of course the treatment of seriously
ill newborns does not always succeed in ensuring
survival, and often, while survival is achieved, permanent disabilities remain. In addition, there remain many congenital defects, such as most forms
of mental retardation, which medicine cannot overcome, even while it may be able to overcome accompanying conditions that threaten survival. Finally,

in many cases the child's prognosis, whether treated or not, is beyond medicine's ability to state with confidence, so that treatment choices must be made without good knowledge of potentially critical facts. For all these reasons, treatment decisions for seriously ill newborns often present difficult ethical problems.

Nonetheless, some cases should be relatively easy. In 1982, in In re Guardianship of Infant Doe, a trial judge in Bloomington, Indiana considered the case of a newborn Downs Syndrome child with intestinal atresia, a relatively unusual congenital defect that occurs much more commonly in Downs Syndrome cases. A blockage in the digestive system renders it impossible for the child to ingest any food, resulting in death by starvation. It is fully remediable with surgery that has relatively low risk, and such surgery is performed routinely on otherwise normal infants. In this case the parents and attending physician agreed to forego the surgery, thus ensuring that the child would die. Their decision was not unprecedented, and indeed an earlier instance of the same decision at Johns Hopkins hospital received considerable attention within the medical community. The Bloomington judge declined to override the parental decision, and the child died before an appeal could be taken. Almost all who have examined this case agree that the judge's decision was wrong.

Intervention to override parental decisions is almost always justified when the child's life is at stake, as it was in Bloomington, particularly when the treatment presents no special risks. The only reason ever offered to refuse corrective surgery was the child's affliction with Down's Syndrome, which causes mental retardation with varying degrees of severity. But if the decision is grounded on the child's own interests, the expected retardation cannot justify nontreatment. There are very severe handicaps for which one might reasonably believe the child himself is better off dead. But Downs Syndrome is not one of them. Many Downs Syndrome children have sufficient ability to benefit from education and training programs, and even to become gainfully employed. Almost all have enough ability to relate to other people and derive pleasure from life. Given this prognosis, the Bloomington "Baby Doe" could be denied the needed corrective surgery only if we believed it appropriate to deny a patient life-saving treatment to accommodate the needs or desires of others. No court has ever embraced such a principle.

Yet we can see why some parents may wish to shed responsibility for the care of a handicapped child, particularly if they have other children whose welfare they worry may be compromised by such responsibilities. This possibility, however, may provide reason to scrutinize parental decisions about handicapped newborns, rather than to defer to them. This is not to deny that responsibility for a seriously ill child can be a crushing burden, depending upon the nature of the child's illness and handicaps, the family's resources, and the needs of other children in the family. But that same problem can

also arise with older children or with adults, and
the involuntary termination of an adult's life-sustaining treatment cannot be justified by advantages
which the patient's death would provide others.
This principle seems inviolate. At the same time,
there are good reasons for the state to assist or even
relieve parents entirely of the burdens of raising a
seriously ill or handicapped child, but existing programs are usually inadequate. In some states a
parent can relinquish their parental rights and
thereby also relieve themselves of all responsibility
for the child's care; programs also exist that subsi-
dize many of the special needs such children have to
make it more possible for the parents to care for
such children themselves. A more comprehensive
array of such options is the proper response to the
plight of these families. Allowing the children to die
is not, except when the death is also in the child's
best interests.

The Bloomington case drew national attention in
1982 when protests by local anti-abortion groups
were sympathetically heard by the Reagan administration, and the phrase "Baby Doe," derived from
the case's caption, became a shorthand label for
seriously ill newborns whose treatment was put in
question. We will shortly consider the federal regulations that resulted. But note first that the Bloomington case itself represents one endpoint on a
continuum of ethically distinguishable possibilities.
The other endpoint can be represented by an anencephalic newborn, a child born with no upper brain.
If it has a functioning brainstem it is still alive. But

no medical procedure is available to correct this gross deformity, which often produces stillbirths and which is typically fatal, regardless of what is done, within weeks of birth. Even apart from its very short lifespan, a child with no upper brain could never develop any self-awareness, much less relate to other human beings. That child's own interests suggest that it is better off with minimal comfort care than with aggressive medical intervention to maximize its lifespan. Although the child will experience no pain in the subjective sense, it may have reflexive reactions to the ordinarily painful stimuli that accompany aggressive medical intervention. And the treatment will confer little benefit on such a child, who is also incapable of deriving any pleasure from the days added to its life.

The case of the anencephalic newborn demonstrates that focusing exclusively on the child's interests is not synonymous with concluding treatment should always be provided. In fact, our deference to the autonomy principle in making similar decisions for adults with decisionmaking capacity is grounded on our understanding that there are indeed occasions when adults will conclude that their self-interest lies in withdrawing treatment. But we also know that not all adults will make the same decision in all cases. Where each can speak for himself, we rely on the autonomy principle to follow the desires of each. But what are we to do in the case of the newborn whose condition and prognosis seem analogous to the kind of case in which different adults might reach different decisions, with regard to their own treatment? That is, what is the proper rule to follow when we are not at either endpoint on the continuum, but in the grey area in between.

We have seen that in the traditional cases of medical neglect, exemplified by *Hofbauer* and *Custody of a Minor,* courts have not been entirely consistent. These two cases involved parents with relatively bizarre treatment preferences, which is typical of medical neglect cases involving older children. For example, the parents may have religious objections to standard medical treatment that almost no parent would otherwise reject. *E.g.,* Hall v. State, 482 N.E.2d 1185 (Ind.App.1985) (child dies from bacterial infection where parents refuse antibiotics on religious grounds); Walker v. Superior Ct., 222 Cal.Rptr. 87 (Cal.App.1986) (same). Such cases present a different dilemma than the newborn cases toward the middle of the ethical continuum, for in the newborn case our hesitation about deferring to a parental decision against treatment comes not from anything unusual about their preferences, but from the simple fact that the child's survival turns on whether we honor them. And pause is surely appropriate when life is in the balance and we have no basis for reliance on an autonomy principle to justify nontreatment. When courts that ordinarily defer to parental treatment decisions hesitate in these circumstances, they act no differently than did the New York courts in dealing with incompetent adult patients in the previously discussed cases of *O'Connor* and *Storar*.

Nonetheless, the arguments in favor of deferring to parental treatment decisions for newborns in these grey area cases is both clear and straightforward: parents ordinarily have full authority to make medical treatment decisions for their children, and we have no basis to override that authority in cases in which reasonable people may differ. The principle might be expressed in this way: In reviewing parental decisions we should not ask whether they made the correct decision, but whether their decision is within the range of decisions that might be made by rational people who are guided entirely by the child's interest. This approach would be consistent with the traditional deference to parental decisions about their children: we do not intrude in parental decisions simply because we disagree. At the same time it appropriately requires that the parents' decision be grounded in the child's interests rather than, for example, the parents' or siblings' interests. We cannot look into the hearts of individual parents to learn their motivations, nor should we adopt the kind of intrusive process that such an inquiry would require. We instead ask whether their decision is one that *could* be made by rational parents concerned exclusively with their child's own interests.

Yet such a principle may be easier to state than to apply. Consider, for example, a child born with spina bifida, a lesion or opening on the back exposing the spinal cord. Such cases vary enormously in prognosis; in many it is clear that full treatment is in the child's interest. But where the lesion is high on the back, and where it is accompanied, as it often is, by hydrocephalus (fluid accumulation in the brain, often causing serious brain damage), the child's prognosis is less favorable. Some such children have additional complications.

The bleakest such cases are very bleak indeed. Attending physicians may conclude that the child has suffered such extensive brain damage that no human social interaction will ever be possible, that the child will never learn to speak, smile, or recognize others. Spinal damage may not only preclude walking, but even sitting up. The aggressive treatment required, both to extend life and to maximize the child's limited potential, may involve numerous surgeries to install shunts in the brain, to repair spinal damage, and to correct other problems. Even with such aggressive treatment, the child's lifespan may be limited, never going much beyond young adulthood. If such a future is known with certainty, it seems clear that a rational person concerned only with the child's welfare could decide that treatment is best declined, thus allowing the child to succumb to an early death. They may plausibly believe that a child with such limited capacity will derive too little benefit from life to make the pain and discomfort of repeated surgery and other intrusive treatment worth enduring. Certainly many if not most adults would choose to decline treatment for themselves, if told they were soon to be in an equivalent situation.

The problem, however, is that medical prognosis is not certain. There is always the hope in such cases that the child will outperform the physician's predictions, as such children sometimes do, and achieve enough capacity to derive real benefit from life. Uncertainty, of course, flows in both directions; children may also do less well than physicians predict. As the physician's ability to predict the child's future becomes less certain, the ethical question becomes more puzzling. People vary in what they are willing to endure to obtain a longer life; they vary as well in how much they would discount the promised additional years by virtue of various disabilities and incapacities. They also vary in their willingness to take risks, which means that the same prediction, when properly couched in terms of *probable* outcome, will be weighed differently by different people on account of their risk-preferences alone. Finally, people may take a different view of the proper way to balance these factors when asked to make a decision for another as opposed to themselves; in particular, they may feel compelled, but in varying degrees, to err in favor of continuing life when confronted with decisions having such uncertain results. The consequence of all these uncertainties is that people disagree strongly not only on what is the best decision, but even on identifying the range of reasonable decisions. In the most difficult cases, what many would find to be the correct decision, others would find entirely outside the range of possible decisions that could be made by a rational person guided entirely by the child's interests.

Judicial resolution of this puzzle was cut short by federal regulation. In 1982 the government announced new rules, issued pursuant to Section 504 of the Rehabilitation Act of 1973, which bars discrimination against the handicapped in programs receiving federal assistance, such as hospitals that accept Medicare or Medicaid patients. The rules barred hospitals from denying medical care to newborn infants on the basis of a handicap. In Bowen v. American Hospital Assoc., 476 U.S. 610 (1986), the Court concluded that the regulations went beyond the intended reach of Section 504, and were therefore void. In the interim, however, Congress dealt with the issue by amending The Child Abuse Prevention and Treatment Act with the Child Abuse Amendments of 1984, P.L. 98–457. As amended the act conditions state receipt of certain federal funds on the state's satisfying legal and administrative criteria to ensure that state child protective agencies will respond, under state child abuse laws, to cases of "medical neglect." 42 U.S.C. § 5106(b)(2)(B). "Medical neglect" is defined to include the "withholding of medically indicated treatment" from disabled infants with "life-threatening conditions." "Medically indicated treatment" is then effectively defined as treatment

> which, in the treating ... physicians' reasonable medical judgment, will be most likely to be effective in ameliorating or correcting all [of the infant's life-threatening] conditions, except that the term does not include the failure to provide treatment ... to an infant when, in the treating physicians' reasonable medical judgment,

(A) the infant is chronically and irreversibly comatose;

(B) the provision of such treatment would (i) merely prolong dying, (ii) not be effective in ameliorating or correcting all of the infant's life threatening conditions, or (iii) otherwise be futile in terms of the survival of the infant; or

(C) the provision of such treatment would be virtually futile in terms of the survival of the infant and the treatment itself under such circumstances would be inhumane.

42 U.S.C. § 5106g(6).

These federal standards are relatively extreme. In general, they appear to require continued treatment in all cases in which life may thereby be extended; the only clear exception is the case of a newborn who is irreversibly comatose. What then of a child, such as those with the most severe cases of spina bifida , for whom life may be extended, but at a cost in pain and discomfort that many would feel is too great to pay for the little pleasure the child will be able to derive from the added years? The last provision, subsection (C), provides the only potential flexibility for allowing discontinuance of treatment in such a case. But that provision seems unlikely to apply, for we probably could not conclude that the treatment would be "virtually futile in terms of the survival of the infant." The statute is subject to some interpretation, of course, but it seems to require continuing any treatment that may extend life by a non-trivial amount. Indeed, upon reflection, the language of this section is quite curious, for it allows the withholding of "inhumane" treatment only when it is "virtually futile" in extending life, implying that even "inhumane" treatment must continue if it may improve the infant's chances of survival. This standard clearly reflects the view that maintaining life is always the overriding concern in treatment decisions. While many have this view, many others do not. Nonetheless, it would seem that if state child abuse authorities are to comply with these federal standards, they will have to restrict considerably the range of discretion that parents are otherwise allowed under traditional rules.

E. DENYING "FUTILE" TREATMENT TO THE PATIENT WHO REQUESTS IT

If the principal of patient autonomy supports the withdrawal of care at the patient's request, what of the patient who *seeks* care that the physician or hospital is otherwise disinclined to provide? This issue, once nearly unheard of, has in recent years become far more important. Advances in medical technology contribute to this result by enlarging the available treatment choices, while changes in medical insurance plans focus attention on the problem. In the era of fee-for-service reimbursement for all treatment, providers had an economic incentive to provide any requested treatment. But where providers are paid on a capitation basis the opposite is true. We are thus more likely to see conflicts in which providers deny treatment that the patient seeks, the mirror image of the traditional ethical dilemma. The general problem is larger than that addressed in this section. Disputes over whether a patient's medical insurance covers an expensive treatment protocol that is nonetheless clearly beneficial for the patient are addressed in chapter 1.D.2, and the general problem of designing medical insurance that allocates resources rationally and ethically is treated in chapter 1.D.1. We here address a more limited but related issue: may a health care provider resist treatment on the grounds that it would confer no medical benefit at all—that the treatment would be *futile*?

On one level the issue seems easy. Every diagnosis necessarily implies a decision to consider some treatments and rule out others. There is no reason to remove the appendix when the diagnosis is stomach flu, and it would be nonsense to argue even that the physician has an ethical duty to discuss the surgical option with the patient, much less to comply with the patient's request for an appendectomy. But other cases are less clear. We might move one step on the implausible-plausible continuum by examining the facts of *Baby K.*, 16 F.3d 590 (4th Cir., 1994), in which the mother sought mechanical breathing assistance for her anencephalic newborn. The baby could breathe on her own for limited periods, and was transferred to a nursing home, but was brought to the hospital emergency room whenever respiratory crises developed. The doctors believed that providing respiratory assistance was medically and ethically inappropriate for a baby with no cerebrum who was on that account doomed to die soon in any event and who, while alive, is permanently unconscious and without the ability to see, hear, think, develop any self-awareness or awareness of her environment. The court nonetheless held the hospital obliged to provide the treatment under EMTALA, an almost certainly unintended result of the legislation that nonetheless follows logically from a mechanical application of its terms. The required breathing assistance was well within the hospital's capabilities and would generally be provided to any emergency room admittee with breathing difficulties, as part of the ordinary and required "stabilization" of the patient's condition. These conclusions, necessary to the court's application of EMTALA, also tell us that while most would agree with the physicians' judgment in this case, that judgment is not based upon the treatment's inability to extend life, and thus the treatment is not literally "futile" in the way that an appendectomy is a futile treatment for stomach flu. The likely consensus on the ethics of this case is instead based upon the view that treatment is inappropriate when it will achieve only a limited extension of life and there is no chance that the life will have any meaning for the patient.

One can thus see that the debate over medical futility is often a debate over values rather than over medical facts. It is thus not usefully resolved by statutes, such as Md. Health Gen. Code § 5–611, that specify that nothing in the law requires "a physician to prescribe or render medically ineffective treatment" (defined in § 601(n) as a medical procedure which, "to a reasonable degree of medical certainty," will not either "(1) Prevent or reduce the deterioration of the health of an individual; or (2) Prevent the impending death of an individual"). Consider, for example, In re Wanglie, 2 BioLaw U:2161 (Aug.-Sept. 1991) (Minn. 4th Dist. Ct.) in which the family sought continued respirator support for an 86 year old diagnosed as irreversibly comatose. Does it matter whether there is some non-zero chance, however slight, that the patient might recover consciousness if kept alive? Does it matter if it is clear that the patient herself wanted to be kept alive, even if comatose, because she valued even that limited an existence?

The same issues arise in connection with Do–Not–Resuscitate (DNR) orders, although the question is often put differently in form because consent to resuscitation is ordinarily presumed. In the case of DNR orders, then, consent is needed to *forego* resuscitation, rather than to provide it, and usual protocols contemplate a discussion of the question between the physician writing the DNR order and the patient or other person who is the patient's medical decisionmaker. The question arises when consent to a DNR order is refused despite the physician's belief that resuscitation would be inappropriate. Consider, for example, In re Jane Doe, 418 S.E.2d 3 (Ga.1992), in which the father refused to consent to a DNR order for his 13 year old daughter, who was suffering from a degenerative nerve disease and "vacillated between stupor and coma". The hospital believed that aggressive medical treatment would constitute abuse, but the court held that state law required the father refuse the order. Resuscitation would thus take place if the girl's heart stopped beating. The court did not consider the futility issue, rendering instead a mechanical application of the state statute. Yet note that if the question were whether to perform surgery for an unrelated condition—imagine, for example, that the girl also developed kidney failure, which might be treated with a transplant from her brother—the physician might simply decide against it without discussion with the parents, and certainly without seeking their permission for the surgery. The statute relied upon in *Doe* would have been inapplicable. Would the physician's decision be ethical? If so, then how does one distinguish the resuscitation required in *Doe*?

DNR orders provide a useful context for discussion of medical futility precisely because the reversal of the usual procedure, requiring permission to *withhold* treatment, highlights the problem. The futility question thus received early attention in the DNR context, with some physicians urging that hospitals allow DNR orders in some cases even without family consultation. A 1988 study found that of 77 hospital patients over 70 who met certain criteria for severity of illness and who were provided CPR, none in fact survived to leave the hospital, although about one-quarter were successfully resuscitated. Schieder & Mayer, *The Decision to Forgo*

CPR in the Elderly Patient, 260 J.A.M.A. 2096 (1988). An accompanying article suggested that it would be permissible to withhold CPR in such cases without first consulting the patient or his family because the treatment was "ineffective." Murphy, *Do Not Resuscitate Orders: Time for Reappraisal in Long–Term Care Institutions,* 260 J.A.M.A. 2098 (1988). More recently the debate has extended to other arenas, as some have argued that physicians are under an ethical duty to all the patients in an insurance pool and should therefore resist requests to "waste" resources on "futile" treatment. And indeed, a survey of intensive care physicians found that 83% reported unilaterally foregoing treatment they believed futile, defined to include treatment that promised no significant chance of "meaningful survival". Asch *et al.,* *Decisions to Limit or Continue Life–Sustaining Treatment by Critical Care Physicians in the United States,* 151 Am.J. Respiratory Critical Care Med. 288 (1995).

Ultimately, it appears that the futility debate may be misnamed. There is little controversy over the small group of cases in which there is true medical futility in the narrow physiological sense, as in our appendectomy example. And the larger group of more difficult cases are not about true medical futility but instead involve value judgments that must share basic principles with the system we adopt generally for allocating health care resources.

CHAPTER 8

SELECTED ISSUES IN
REPRODUCTIVE
MEDICINE

A. ASSISTED CONCEPTION

After making it convenient to have sex without conception, science made it possible to have conception without sex. It then became necessary to revisit traditional legal rules attributing parentage, and to consider new rules establishing the status of fertilized human eggs, (and their immediate descendant, multi-cell human "embryos" at a pre-implantation stage), which can now exist outside the body of any human female. These are the topics we address in this part of the Chapter.

1. Artificial Insemination by Donor (Aid)

a. Basic Rules

Artificial insemination is an older medical procedure whose availability long predates the modern cases that have drawn most of the public attention to assisted conception issues. It is traditionally employed by married women with infertile husbands. When they are impregnated artificially with a donor's sperm, state law typically provides that the woman's husband, not the sperm donor, is the child's legal father, either by case law (People v. Sorensen, 437 P.2d 495 (Cal.1968)) or by statute (see § 5 of the Uniform Parentage Act). (We ignore cases in which the husband's sperm is used, as they raise no issues of parentage attribution.)

Today's interesting cases often involve new uses of this older technology. For example, the Uniform Parentage Act (U.P.A.) simply does not address the case of an artificially-impregnated woman with no husband to whom the law may assign paternal responsibilities. Is the sperm donor then the legal father, or is there no legal father? Several adopting states omit the limitation to "married" women from the U.P.A. rule that the sperm donor is not the legal father. Their versions of the U.P.A. thus appear to leave no man with paternal rights or responsibilities to the AID child of an unmarried woman. In cases involving unmarried women, however, courts in those states have sometimes held that the sperm donor is the child's legal father when either: a) no physician is involved in the insemination, (Jhordan C. v. Mary K., 224 Cal.Rptr. 530 (App. 1986) and C.O. v. W.S., 639 N.E.2d 523 (Ohio Com.Pleas, 1994)); or b) when the mother and donor agreed beforehand that the donor would be the father (In re R.C., 775 P.2d 27 (Colo.1989) (remanded to determine whether parties made such an agreement, as the donor alleged)). But this approach is not universal. McIntyre v. Crouch, 780 P.2d 239 (Or.App.1989) (divided court finds semen donor is not the father under statutory rule even though mother was single, performed insemination on herself without physician's assistance, and knew donor, but that the rule's application to this case would violate the federal constitution if donor had agreement with mother that he would act as the child's father).

b. Use by Lesbian Couples

In many of the AID cases involving an unmarried woman, the mother is part of a lesbian couple who intend to raise the resulting child together, and who do not wish the sperm donor to have a parental relationship with the child. They sometimes have an explicit agreement to that effect with the donor. Prevailing law, however, often denies enforcement to such pre-birth disavowals of parenthood, and sometimes the lesbian couple themselves undercut the agreement by permitting the donor contact with the child. Whether because of this contact (Thomas v. Robin, 618 N.Y.S.2d 356 (App.Div.1994) (donor recognized as father where he had social relationship with the child)) or as a result of the rules already surveyed, *Jhordan C., supra*, donors in such cases are sometimes recognized as the child's father despite the parties' agreement. However, when the AID is carried out with the assistance of medical personnel, and particularly when the donor is anonymous, the child will usually have no legally recognized father. Perhaps for this reason among others, medical personnel traditionally declined to perform inseminations of unmarried women, and a 1988 study found that 61 percent of physicians said they would reject requests for AID from an unmarried woman "without a partner." Of course, a legally unmarried lesbian woman may well have a partner, and today many succeed in becoming pregnant under circumstances excluding recognition of any legal father.

For these lesbian couples, the pressing question is often whether the mother's partner will be recognized in the law as a parent of the resulting child. Adoption is the conventional method for establishing a legally recognized parental relationship with a child who is not biologically related. The recent trend strongly favors petitions by the mother and her partner for adoption of the child by the partner. The normal consequence is that the child has two legally recognized mothers, and no legally recognized father. See, e.g., Adoption of Galen, 680 N.E.2d 70 (Mass.1997). There is one recent state high court decision to the contrary, Interest of Angel, 516 N.W.2d 678 (Wis.1994). Interestingly, Scandanavian countries, which have otherwise been more open than American states to recognition of same-sex marriage, reject adoption by same-sex couples. See Ellman, Kurtz and Scott, FAMILY LAW: CASES, TEXT, PROBLEMS 1128–1130 (3d. ed., 1998). Where there has been no adoption and the lesbian relationship later dissolves, courts are not usually receptive to claims by the mother's former partner for access to the child over the mother's objection, although a few have been.

2. Surrogate Motherhood, Egg Donation, and In–Vitro Fertilization

In a traditional simple egg donation, an otherwise normal woman who is incapable of producing fertile eggs can nonetheless become pregnant with her husband's child, by using his sperm to fertilize a donated egg *in-vitro* ("in glass", meaning in the laboratory rather than within the female's body), before implantation in her uterus. This process is analogous to classic AID, which allows an infertile man to be the legal father of a child born to his wife. Surrogate motherhood describes a relationship rather than any single method or a technology, and may or may not employ egg donation. The relationship is one in which a woman, called the surrogate mother, gestates a child who, by the parties' prior agreement, is intended to be the child of another woman—called the intended mother or, more simply, the mother. In the original and simplest form of surrogate motherhood, the child is the genetic child of the surrogate, who has typically become impregnated through artificial insemination using the sperm of the intended mother's husband. In a more recent variation, an egg from the intended mother is fertilized in-vitro, typically with the sperm of her husband, and then implanted in the surrogate's uterus. The technologies of egg harvesting, in-vitro fertilization, and implantation thus permit complete separation of the identities of sperm donor, egg donor, gestational mother, and intended mother and father, so that up to five persons, all possibly unmarried, can have some relationship to the resulting child.

a. *Surrogacy Contracts Under Traditional Law*

While traditional law clearly did not contemplate such surrogate arrangements, many existing principles seem to bear on them. Most of the potentially applicable law comes from the field of adoption, and poses barriers to the enforcement of any contract between the surrogate and the intended adoptive mother.

(1) Regulation of Private Placement Adoptions. Most American states allow "private placement" adoptions in which the biological parents make arrangements with the adoptive parents themselves, either directly or through an intermediary such as a lawyer. A judicial proceeding is still required to formalize the adoption and establish the adoptive parents' rights, and in that proceeding the judge will receive evidence to establish that the adoptive parents meet required standards of fitness. In addition, most states regulate any payments made by the adoptive parents, either to the biological mother who relinquishes her child for adoption, or to the lawyer or other intermediary. The details of these laws vary, as to both substance and procedure, but most share a common theme. Intermediaries may not collect fees for securing the child or the mother's consent; this means, for example, that an attorney intermediary may collect fees for actual legal work done, but not for services as a child broker. E.g., Galison v. District of Columbia, 402 A.2d 1263 (D.C.App.1979). Biological mothers may be compensated for expenses they incur as a result of the pregnancy, such as medical bills and, depending upon the details of state regulation, possibly lost earnings or basic living expenses, but they may not be paid a fee in exchange for their consent to the

adoption. Such a fee might be considered unlawful baby-selling.

It is clear that such rules pose potential problems for the classic surrogacy contract, in which the surrogate bears a child conceived through artificial insemination using the sperm of the intended mother's husband. The fee paid to the surrogate is, in part, payment for the consent to adopt, even though it is also compensation for undergoing the pregnancy and delivery. That is clear because the intended mother enters the agreement in order to receive the child for adoption, and often final payments are not made until custody is transferred to her and her husband. The willingness of the surrogate to permit her adoption of the child is therefore an essential part of the agreement. The fee promised by the agreement may thus be illegal. In some states all fee arrangements made in connection with an adoption must be disclosed in the adoption proceedings and approved by the court; clearly fees paid in exchange for the consent would not be approved.

The requirement that a court review and approve the fitness of the adoptive parents means that completion of the adoption is not entirely in the parties' control. However, as implemented in most private placement adoptions, this process would not usually cause a problem so long as the parties remain in agreement, because the court's evaluation of the adoptive parents is not ordinarily comparative: The court does not ask whether better parents could be found for the child, but only whether these parents are acceptable, and most intended adoptive mothers under surrogacy agreements surely meet this test. Nonetheless, the surrogate contract arrangement might not work to provide a child to a mother who is clearly unsuitable. Moreover, if the parties do not remain in agreement, the surrogate, as the legal mother at birth, will have priority over the intended mother. Most states do not recognize consent to adoption given by the mother prior to the birth of the child. The surrogate mother is thus free to repudiate any consent to adoption she may have given in the pre-birth surrogate contract.

(2) Rights and Identity of the Father. While the surrogate may be able to repudiate the consent to adoption of her child that she gave in a surrogacy contract, she cannot thereby exclude claims by the father of her child. In such a case, if the father promptly asserts his rights, he will transform the dispute into an ordinary custody contest. Given the relative situations of the typical surrogate and the typical father, one might expect the father to win such contests most of the time. The father usually has a stable marriage; the mother may not be married. The father is typically financially secure, as the cost of surrogate agreements for the adoptive parents will usually exclude those who are not; the mother is often financially insecure, which may be why she agreed to serve as a surrogate mother in the first place. The differences in economic status will usually be correlated with differences in educational attainments and employment status, with the result that the father's overall situation will be more favorable for the child than the mother's.

One possible difficulty for the father may arise from the rules governing AID, reviewed above, under which the surrogate's husband, if she has one, rather than the semen donor, might be considered the legal father of the surrogate's child. To forestall such results, surrogacy agencies typically require the written agreement of the surrogate's husband, where she has one, but the legal effect of such agreements has not been tested. Of course, AID statutes were not written with surrogacy agreements in mind, and a court might therefore choose not to apply the statute to such a case.

(3) *In re* Baby M. The difficulties of enforcing surrogacy contracts under traditional law is well illustrated by an early but still well-known surrogate mothering case, In re Baby M, 537 A.2d 1227 (N.J.1988). Elizabeth Stern, a physician, determined that she had multiple sclerosis, and was unwilling to go through a pregnancy because of the risk to her health which she believed would result. Nonetheless, she and her husband, William Stern, wanted children. William contracted with Mary Beth Whitehead to bear his child, the two having been brought together by the Infertility Center of New York, which specialized in finding surrogate mothers for infertile couples. Whitehead was married and had children. She had previously offered to be a surrogate for another couple, but never became pregnant. Artificial insemination with Mr. Stern's sperm was successful, however. After the child was born, Whitehead had great doubts about her ability to surrender it; among other things, she felt the

child closely resembled her other daughter. Despite her doubts she surrendered the child to the Sterns three days after the birth. But that evening she called the Sterns in despair. Afraid that Whitehead might commit suicide if she did not see the child again, the Sterns agreed to return her to Whitehead for a week.

In fact, the Sterns did not recover the baby until four months later, when she was forcibly removed from Whitehead's parents' home in Florida, to which Mary Beth had fled with the child. From that time forward, Melissa, as the Sterns called her, lived with the Sterns, while a court battle over her ensued. The Sterns sought enforcement of the surrogacy contract; they also alleged that the child's best interests supported placing her with them.

The contract had three parties: William Stern, Mary Whitehead, and Mary's husband, Richard. Mary had agreed to become pregnant, carry the child, bear it, deliver it to the Sterns, and do whatever was necessary to terminate her parental rights so that Elizabeth Stern could adopt the child. Richard promised to do whatever was necessary to rebut the presumption of his paternity that would arise under New Jersey law, since the child would be born to his wife. Mr. Stern agreed to pay Mary Beth $10,000 upon delivery of the child to him, and also to pay the Infertility Center $7500 for its services, which were to include completing the adoption process. Elizabeth was not a party to the agreement, but it provided that in the event of William's death she would have sole custody.

The court concluded that while all parties had entered the agreement in good faith, it was not enforceable under New Jersey law. The specified payments to both Whitehead and the Infertility Center were found to violate New Jersey statutes regulating the fees that could be charged in connection with adoption. The court rejected the claim that the fees to Whitehead were only for "services," concluding instead that they were prohibited payments for her consent to Elizabeth's adoption of the child, and it rejected the claim that the fees paid to the Infertility Center were only for legal services. In reaching these conclusions the court looked beyond the characterization of these payments contained in the agreement, focusing instead on what it viewed as the reality of the exchange.

The court also found that an agreement to surrender a child not yet born was not enforceable under New Jersey law because it did not comply with any of the permissible New Jersey procedures under which parental rights can be terminated. "[A] contractual agreement to abandon one's parental rights, or not to contest a termination action, will not be enforced in our courts." *Id*. at 1243. If Whitehead's parental rights were not terminated, then the adoption could not go forward. It also found that there was nothing in the record that would justify an involuntary termination of Whitehead's parental rights, given the well established family law principle that a parent's rights cannot be terminated merely because a court judges that a better parent is available. A parent whose fitness meets minimum standards has a protected interest in retaining her parental rights as against a stranger, even one who seems superior.

With the contract effectively voided, the case turned into a custody contest between the girl's legally recognized parents, Mr. Stern and Mrs. Whitehead. The court held that the contest should be judged by the traditional custody decision rule: placement is determined by the child's best interests, giving no weight to the surrogacy contract. In comparing the Whitehead and Stern homes, the court found, not surprisingly, that the evidence strongly favored the Stern's. While granting Mr. Stern primary custody, the court also held that Mary Beth Whitehead was entitled to visitation rights, a result which followed almost necessarily from their decision that her parental rights continue. The trial court later ruled that Whitehead would be entitled to 8 hours of unsupervised visitation per week, to increase over the course of the year to two days every two weeks, including overnight.

Baby M. is a straightforward application of traditional rules. While its analysis was followed by most courts, at least one held that the anti-baby selling provisions contained in adoption and custody laws were not intended to apply to surrogacy arrangements, and thus did not bar surrogacy contracts. Surrogate Parenting Associates v. Kentucky, 704 S.W.2d 209 (Ky.1986). Note also that most surrogate parenting contracts are carried out successfully, in that the parties do not later disagree, and for them the refusal of courts to enforce the agreement

may not matter. Even then, however, to complete
their intended transaction, the surrogate will have
to execute, post-birth, a document relinquishing her
parental rights, and judicial approval of the intended mother's adoption will be required. But even if
the surrogacy contract is not valid in the sense that
it would not be enforced over the surrogate's objection, where there is no objection courts are likely to
approve the adoption despite the fact that the
child's existence results from the invalid contract.
E.g., Adoption of Baby A and Baby B, 877 P.2d 107
(Or. App.1994).

There was considerable legislative activity after
Baby M., and today nearly half the states have
statutes regulating surrogacy agreements. Only a
few criminalize the making of such agreements;
most simply declare the contract void, a result consistent with traditional law. A handful recognize
surrogacy contracts, but most of these combine that
recognition with important limitations, such as dis-
allowing payments to the surrogate that exceed her
expenses, or allowing the surrogate to revoke her
agreement and keep the child if she acts promptly
after birth. The most accepting state statute is
probably Virginia's, which allows enforcement of
surrogacy agreements that meet a host of regulatory requirements. It is based upon the permissive
alternative, offered to states that wish to allow
surrogacy, contained in the Uniform Status of Children of Assisted Conception Act. For a more complete description of the various state laws, see Ell-

man, Kurtz and Scott, FAMILY LAW: CASES, TEXT, PROBLEMS 1498–99 (3d ed., 1998).

b. Gestational Surrogacy and Changing Law

Whether or not one believes it invokes the appropriate policy, the traditional law applied in *Baby M.* yields a clear result where the surrogate is the biological mother of the child in question. More confused, however, is the case in which the surrogate is the child's gestational mother but the intended mother is also the child's genetic mother. This occurs when a fertilized egg of the intended mother is implanted in the uterus of the surrogate, who then carries the child to term. In the event of a dispute, which woman should the law recognize as the child's legal mother? Under these facts one is tempted to conclude that the genetic mother should prevail. Yet consider the equally possible case in which the gestational mother is the intended mother—where, unable to produce her own fertile eggs, she carries to term a donated egg that was fertilized in-vitro with her husband's sperm. Should the egg donor then be able to claim the child is hers?

Faced with such possibilities, the California Supreme Court concluded that both gestational and genetic mothers satisfy the traditional legal standards for "mother" contained in statutes like the Uniform Parentage Act, since motherhood under those pre-technology standards could be shown by either genetic proof or by evidence of having given birth to the child. Declining to give both women the status of legal mother, the court concluded that the question should be decided according to the intent of the parties at the time of the child's conception. It therefore held that the surrogate, who in the case before it had carried to term the intended mother's genetic child, was not the child's legal mother, and must therefore surrender it to the intended mother and her husband (whose sperm had been used to fertilize his wife's egg in-vitro). Johnson v. Calvert, 851 P.2d 776 (Cal.1993).

If the parties' intent had been the test applied in *Baby M.*, then the surrogacy contract there would have been effectively enforceable. But California has not applied the *Johnson* intent test to traditional surrogacies of the *Baby M.* kind. See Moschetta v. Moschetta, 30 Cal.Rptr. 2d 893 (App. 1994) (holding that the intent of the parties was relevant only when the gestational mother is not the genetic mother, and that surrogacy agreement could not therefore be enforced over the opposition of surrogate who was both the gestational and genetic mother). On the other hand, the intent test was employed in a relatively bizarre case at the other extreme. In Buzzanca v. Buzzanca, 72 Cal.Rptr.2d 280 (App. 1998) the parties, while married, had a fertilized egg implanted in the uterus of a surrogate who had agreed to carry the child to term. Neither husband nor wife was genetically related to the child. When husband and wife filed for divorce before the child's birth, the court had to decide whether this was a child "of the marriage". The husband denied all rights and responsibility to the child, as did its gestational mother. The wife asserted she was the child's legal mother, and claimed primary custody as well as child support from her husband as its legal father. The genetic parents were not parties to the case and were apparently unknown. The trial court reached the "extraordinary" conclusion, as the appeals court put it, that the child had no legal parents. Reversing, the appeals court applied *Johnson* by analogy to conclude that husband and wife were the child's lawful parents.

A complete survey of the ethical and moral debates that still rage over surrogacy is beyond the scope of this book. The most willing defense of the practice comes from those who view public policy issues economically. *See* Richard Epstein, *Surrogacy: The Case for Full Contractual Enforcement*, 81 Va.L.Rev. 2305 (1995); Richard Posner, *The Ethics and Economics of Enforcing Contracts of Surrogate Motherhood*, 5 J.Contemp.Health L. & Pol. 21 (1989). John Robertson, in CHILDREN OF CHOICE (1994), argues that the Constitutional right of privacy should protect the right to enter and enforce surrogacy contracts, as a form of "non-coital" reproduction. Robertson, . Some argue against surrogacy contracts on the grounds that they are harmful to children. Margaret Brinig, *A Materialistic Approach to Surrogacy: A Comment on Richard Epstein's Surrogacy*, 81 Va.L.Rev. 2377 (1995). Other well-known commentators on this topic include Martha Field, SURROGATE MOTHERHOOD (1988) and Marjorie Shultz, *Reproductive Technology and Intent–Based Parenthood*, 1990 Wisc.L.Rev. 297, whose views were in part the basis of the California Supreme Court's analysis in *Calvert*. Feminists have been of two minds. Some believe that allowing surrogate motherhood is consistent with ensuring all women full individual freedom of choice in making use of their own reproductive capacities. Lori Andrews, *Surrogate Motherhood: The Challenge for Feminists,* 16 L.Med. & Health Care 78 (1988) (surrogacy is a "predictable outgrowth of the feminist movement"). Others worry about the commodification of women's reproductive capacities. E. Anderson, Value in Ethics and Economics 168–190 (1993); Margaret J. Radin, Contested Commodities (1996). See also D. Callahan, *No Child Wants to Live in a Womb for Hire,* Nat'l Catholic Reporter, October 11, 1985 ("Women object to being baby factories or sex objects because it offends their human dignity."). One well–known ethicist has condemned surrogacy as baby-selling, the moral equivalent of slavery, George Annas, *Fairy Tales Surrogate Mothers Tell,* 16 L.Med. & Health Care 27 (1988). The Catholic Church, not surprisingly, has condemned surrogate motherhood on the basis of its belief that sex and reproduction cannot be uncoupled and cannot take place outside of marriage.

3. The Status of Stored Embryos

There are a variety of medical conditions which leave a woman unable to become pregnant even though she has healthy eggs and a functioning uterus that would allow her to carry the child if she became pregnant. For example, a problem in the

fallopian tubes may disrupt the normal movement
of the eggs from the ovaries. In-vitro fertilization
may be an effective fertility treatment in such
cases. The woman's egg is removed, fertilized in-
vitro with her partner's sperm, allowed divide to
the four-or eight-cell stage, and then transferred to
the woman's uterus with a cervical catheter. If this
"embryo" attaches to the uterine wall, a normal
pregnancy may result. This procedure does not normally produce parentage issues, since the woman
who bears the child is also its genetic and intended
mother, and in the usual case the genetic father is
the mother's husband. The difficulty of harvesting
eggs for such a procedure, however, yields another
potential problem. To spare the woman the experience of repeated harvestings, IVF programs typically harvest multiple eggs at one time, which may
then all be fertilized. These embryos may be preserved in liquid nitrogen, available for implantation
at a later date. What if that later date never comes?
Couples who have achieved a successful pregnancy
using IVF may choose to donate their "spare"
embryos to another infertile couple, but it seems
that most choose to retain them for possible future
pregnancies. But what if the couple cannot agree?

In Davis v. Davis, 842 S.W.2d 588 (Tenn.1992), a
divorcing couple had seven frozen embryos in stor-
age at a Knoxville fertility clinic where they had
sought, unsuccessfully, to achieve a viable pregnancy. When the parties first sought divorce the wife
wished to continue her attempts to become pregnant through post-divorce implantation of the

embryos, to which the husband objected. By the time the matter came to the state high court for review, both parties had remarried. She now wanted to donate the embryos for use by another couple, while he had become quite firm in opposing any procedure that would result in the birth of a child. The trial court, in a bizarre decision, treated the matter as a child custody dispute and awarded "custody" of the four-cell embryos to the wife. While rejecting this characterization of the issue, the state high court also declined to embrace a rule automatically requiring approval of both progenitors before implantation could take place, an approach that would have necessarily vindicated the husband's position. The court instead concluded that the decision in such cases required balancing the interests of the particular parties in the case as they had expressed them.

Mr. Davis was said to strongly oppose fathering any child who would not live with both its parents, while his former wife's desire to donate the embryos was said to be based on her desire to make some use of the embryos after having gone through the lengthy IVF procedures. The court concluded that her interest in donation was less weighty than his in avoiding parenthood. Moreover, while agreeing that her interest would have been stronger had she sought to use the embryos herself, the court also suggested that it would still have been insufficient. Thus, while in form avoiding any bright line rules, the court's approach toward balancing would in most if not all cases seem to favor the party opposing use of the embryos. The court did leave open the possibility, however, that it might have decided this case in the wife's favor had use of these embryos been her only chance to bear her own children, particularly if she had not previously expressed a willingness to consider adoption.

In reaching its result, the *Davis* court noted that the parties had no prior agreement concerning the disposition of the embryos. It indicated that if they had made such an agreement at the time they arranged for the IVF procedures, the agreement should be enforced (unless, of course, the parties later agreed to some other result). It appears that most IVF programs now routinely require participants to indicate on their consent forms how they wish to handle unused embryos. In Kass v. Kass, 91 N.Y.2d 554 (N.Y. 1998), the consent form contained a section in which the parties could choose, from a provided list of alternatives, the disposition they preferred "[i]n the event that we ... are unable to make a decision regarding the disposition of our stored, frozen pre-zygotes." The Kasses chose: "Our frozen pre-zygotes may be examined by the IVF Program for biological studies and be disposed of by the IVF Program for approved research investigation as determined by the IVF Program." When the parties later divorced, the wife wanted to attempt post-divorce implantation with their five frozen pre-embryos, claiming that it was her only chance for genetic parenthood. Her former husband objected, and he prevailed when New York held that the executed consent form constituted an enforceable agreement between them on the matter which governed this dispute.

4. Genetic Medicine

Modern genetic research allows medical science to move beyond merely facilitating the fact of conception, to altering, and presumably improving, its product. No regular newspaper reader can be unaware of the frequent articles announcing the discovery of a gene for this or that disease, and perhaps many would not be surprised to read that scientists had found the gene for high LSAT scores or for playing a jazz trumpet. But genetics is more complex than that. Nearly every human trait of interest is affected by many different genes, as well as by the environment with which they interact. It matters little to be genetically lactose-intolerant in a culture that consumes no dairy products, and aptitude for higher mathematics may not be discernable in a culture with no schools.

But while these cautions need be kept in mind, there is no denying that we are in the midst of an explosion of knowledge about human genetics that must have social as well as scientific implications. The Human Genome Project, an enormous research program involving scientists in dozens of locations, will, in the not-distant future, generate a complete map of the human genome. The next step, far more complex, lies in understanding the function of each gene. Many are of course already understood, and prenatal diagnosis for a number of genetic diseases is already well-established. (Early prenatal diagnosis of full-chromosome abnormalities, such as Down's Syndrome, has been established for quite some time, as has the ability to learn the sex of a fetus, but detecting abnormalities in individual genes has been achieved only in recent years.) Genetic tests are also emerging that predict future health problems for adults, such as cancer or neurological disorders.

What shall we do with such knowledge? There are many applications and implications beyond the scope of this chapter, such as genetic screening by health and life insurers, and the possibilities for marketing laboratory-made genetic material and for claiming ownership of genetic processes and structures. Here, we describe briefly only the possible uses of genetic technologies that are related to the reproduction issues surveyed in this chapter. We first consider the possibility that individuals may be offered the chance to learn whether they are afflicted with, or carriers of, known genetic diseases.

Let us start with the fairly straightforward example of Huntington's Chorea, sometimes known as Woody Guthrie disease. This neurological disease leads to impaired motor control, involuntary muscular contractions, personality changes, and dementia. The defective gene is dominant, so there is no distinction between carrier and sufferer—a single gene, inherited from either parent, produces the affliction. The disease, while devastating, does not typically emerge until well into adulthood, giving the affected person plenty of time to bear children of his or her own—each with a 50% chance of inheriting the disease. So Alice might learn, at age 25, for example, that one of her parents has Huntington's. Just a decade ago the result was uncertainty. Alice knew she had a fifty percent chance herself, but she might not yet show symptoms, even if she had the gene, since onset typically occurs between the ages of 30 and 50. Today genetic testing is available. Not every potential Huntington's sufferer has sought to be tested. Some prefer to remain uncertain rather than risk confirmation that they are affected. But then should such a person herself have children? If she is afflicted, half her children, on average, will be as well. Some believe it is not ethical to bear children knowing of their potential suffering—and of the possibility that their parent will not survive to their adulthood.

Of course, prenatal diagnosis may be available. Even if Alice is generally comfortable with having an abortion to avoid bearing a child with serious genetic defects, is it a different matter for her to become pregnant knowing her heightened risk for that result? If so, is in-vitro fertilization a choice? That is, Alice could have her eggs harvested, have them fertilized in-vitro, and then have them examined for presence of the Huntington's gene—and go forward with the implantation only of a zygote without Huntington's.

Indeed, the ability to do pre-implantation genetic examination raises other possibilities. Some genetic diseases are treatable with transplants from genetically compatible relatives. An inherited anemia, for example, might be treatable with a bone marrow transplant from a healthy sibling. Of course, the sibling might also be affected by the same disease. There are reports that some parents of children afflicted with an otherwise fatal anemia have had additional children in the hope of producing a child who can serve as a life-saving donor for their sibling. Yet the chance of a child who is both healthy and genetically compatible is only 1 in 4. These parents, feeling under pressure to produce a healthy donor in time to save their existing child, might choose to become pregnant, obtain prenatal diagnosis, and then abort if the resulting baby could not be a donor, in order to quickly try again. But IVF technology makes this drastic and controversial measure unnecessary, for these parents now can instead test which of several zygotes to implant in order to produce a healthy marrow donor.

Techniques like these, which are only now beginning to emerge, are limited only by the current state of genetic knowledge. At some point scientists may be able to look at the zygotes available for IVF and distinguish those with higher probabilities of being smart, tall, or blond from those with lower probabilities for those traits. Should such knowledge be available for clinical application? If adults may choose to have purely cosmetic surgery, should they also be allowed to choose zygotes whose genes give their children an improved chance for maturing into more attractive adults? Needless to say, these questions do not now have legal answers, but at some point they probably will. Or, these issues may be forestalled by legal obstacles placed in the path of technology development that seems too threatening to social values. For example, the federal government refuses to fund research using fetal tissue because of the concern this might create a market for abortions. More recently, the 1997 announcement by a British scientist that he had produced a genetic clone of a sheep named Dolly has led to calls for banning or refusing to fund studies directed toward cloning humans.

It is sometimes thought that, while it is possible to alter or control genetic makeup prior to birth, you are stuck with whatever genes you have when you are born, but this is no longer true. At the end of 1994, there were over 100 approved clinical protocols offering gene therapy—therapeutic interventions that alter the existing genetic structure in patients suffering various genetically affected diseases. These are still experimental protocols, but at some point they will lead to generally approved treatments that will be widely available. The issue raised in the preceding paragraph is no different in principle from those raised by gene therapy. Suppose gene therapy were available to improve the cognitive function of those congenitally afflicted with mental handicaps, such as sufferers of Downs Syndrome. If we are willing to modify the structure or functions of their genes to improve their cognitive functioning, would we refuse to allow a different gene therapy that would improve the cognitive functioning of those whose intelligence is in the "normal" range?

Finally, there is the possibility of preventive genetic medicine, through the use of genetic screening. Indeed, one might imagine mandatory genetic testing whose purpose is to inform individuals about important aspects of their own genes. For example, some people dramatically raise their chance of suffering a heart attack if they eat a high fat diet, while others are immune to such effects. Both would likely find it useful to know which they are. Perhaps even more intriguing is the possibility of learning the particular genetic traits one might wish to seek or avoid in a mate. Many genetic diseases result from recessive genes. The person with only one may experience no important deleterious impact, because the normal other gene is dominant. But the child who inherits the defective gene from each of his parents is seriously afflicted. It may seem advisable for people who share recessive genes for the same genetic disease to avoid having children together, for one of every four of their children will suffer the defect, and another two will (like them) be a carrier for it. Other alternatives for them include prenatal genetic tests, perhaps followed by abortion, or in-vitro fertilization in which zygotes who are homozygous for the recessive gene are discarded.

The choice among these alternatives depends on one's values, but any of the choices is facilitated by knowledge that special risks are associated with these two particular people having children together. The chance that two randomly chosen people from the population will share such deleterious defective genes is generally remote, but people do not choose their mates randomly from the population. They are indeed more likely to marry within their own ethnic group, and most ethnic groups have a heightened frequency of some genetic diseases (and a lowered frequency of others). For example, Tay–Sachs disease, while generally rare, occurs much more frequently among Jews of Eastern European ancestry than among the population at large, and sickle cell anemia is much more common among those of African ancestry.

There are not yet any general programs to test individuals for dangerous recessive genes, in part due to the high costs involved, but this may soon change. Currently, debate focuses on whether there should be widespread genetic screening for carriers of the cystic fibrosis gene, in order to inform couples who both have this recessive trait that they are at 1–in–4 risk of having affected children. This remains controversial because of the costs relative to the low incidence of the disease in the general population (about 1 in 1000) and because the test has a significant false negative rate (that is, it misses a large number of actual carriers because not all of the mutations are known).

More feasible are programs targeted at specific high risk subgroups where testing is more full-proof. Tightly knit subcultures in which marriages with outsiders are rare are particularly good candidates for community-wide programs that test for all genes for which that group is at high risk. And indeed, one such group in New York routinely tests all children of one sex. Arranged marriages are the norm in this group. Confidential records are kept of children who are found in these routine tests to have a deleterious recessive gene. When a marriage is proposed for that child, the intended mate is tested, and if the mate shares the trait, community leaders advise the proposed couple's families against the marriage, on the ground that the couple is "genetically incompatible." If such a program can work today in an appropriate subgroup, perhaps advancing technology will someday lower costs sufficiently to make it financially practical to propose more generally.

These issues are complex and at this point often speculative, and so we only touch upon them here. While it may be possible to respond adequately to a number of these issues with existing legal rules, many of these advances in genetic technology are sure to pose fundamental challenges and expose serious weaknesses in the existing legal structure.

B. MATERNAL–FETAL CONFLICT

From conception to childbirth the lives of the mother and her unborn child have a biological and psychological connection that is unique. Medicine traditionally focused its attentions on the mother, having little it could offer to improve the child's prospects other than keeping the mother in good health. The unborn child was not accessible to the doctor, and thus could not be treated as a separate patient with his own needs.[1] But over the past few decades this has become less true, for two reasons. First, we have much more information today about the effect on fetal health of particular maternal behaviors such as smoking, drinking, or using drugs. Second, physicians have a much greater ability to intervene with procedures directed expressly at fetal health, but which require treatment of the mother as well in order to reach the fetus. A new ethical puzzle has thereby been created: to what extent, if any, is the mother ethically or legally obligated to follow medical advice reasonably thought necessary to protect the health of her child?

This section divides maternal-fetal conflict cases into two categories, depending upon whether the contested medical advice involves surgery. The most common surgical procedure recommended for fetal health is delivery by Caesarean section. In recent years physicians have also developed techniques to perform surgery on the fetus in-utero, a process which of course also requires surgery on the mother.

The discussion that follows assumes the continued existence of a woman's right to abort, at least in the early stages of pregnancy. The general subject of abortion is too large to cover in this volume, particularly as it is treated fully elsewhere. But in any event the ethical and legal issues posed by

1. For ease of expression, throughout this section the child will be referred to with the masculine pronoun, to distinguish him from the mother.

maternal-fetal conflicts are not entirely the same as those posed by abortion, and a separate analysis is therefore required in any event. We will see that appropriate resolution of these matters need not turn on one's position in the abortion debate. On one hand, there is no necessary inconsistency in combining a public policy that recognizes a woman's right to terminate her pregnancy, with another policy that imposes obligations on her with respect to the conduct of her pregnancy *if* she chooses to continue it to term. On the other hand, we will see that in at least some of the cases, the fetus can be aided only if we impose on the pregnant woman a more onerous burden than that which the law would require of her with regard to her born children. In those cases we might reject imposing such duties on her even if we believe that the fetus is the full moral equivalent of the born child and that abortion should be unlawful.

1. Forced Caesareans and Fetal Surgery

The proportion of all childbirths in the U.S. that are by Cesarean increased from about five percent in the mid 1960's to about 25 percent in 1988. This increase is at least in part the result of a significant decline, over the same period of time, in the risk that Caesarian section poses to the mother. For example, the maternal mortality rate for Caesareans in 1970 was nearly three times the 1978 rate of one in 2500. The procedure's increased safety means that, more often than before, it is a less risky method of childbirth for the mother herself. Of greater importance for our discussion is the fact that the procedure's increased safety makes the physician more inclined to recommend it in cases where vaginal delivery poses a risk to the child's health. Thus, Caesareans are an important example of newfound physician ability to intervene directly to preserve the child's health through procedures that necessarily intrude on the mother. What is the appropriate legal response if the mother refuses to consent to the intrusion?

The issue first received widespread attention in the 1980's, when a survey of obstetrical residency programs found a fair number of cases in which physicians had obtained, in unreported trial court decisions, orders compelling women to submit to Caesareans thought necessary to their child's survival. The early appellate decisions were not precisely on point, but seemed to support these trial courts. Some involved Jehovah's Witnesses who consented to Caesarean sections but not to blood transfusions. Because transfusions may become necessary during any surgical procedure, surgeons generally insist upon authorization for them before proceeding with any surgery. Two of these cases held that the woman could be compelled to accept the transfusions where the Caesarean was thought essential to her child's survival. Jefferson v. Griffin Spalding County Hospital Authority, 274 S.E.2d 457 (Ga.1981); Raleigh Fitkin–Paul Morgan Mem. Hosp. v. Anderson, 201 A.2d 537 (N.J.1964). Arrayed against this meager but vaguely supportive authority was the almost universal criticism of commentators. *E.g.,* Nancy Rhoden, *The Judge in the Delivery Room: Emergence of Court–Ordered Caesareans,* 74 Calif.L.Rev. 1951 (1986). In 1987, the Committee on Ethics of the American College of Obstetricians and Gynecologists concluded that resort to the courts in cases where the patient rejects the physician's advice "is almost never warranted" and "violates the pregnant woman's autonomy."

The initial reaction of the courts was not surprising. Where the physician claims that the baby will die imminently without a Caesarean, the trial judge, who typically needs to make a decision on the spot, will surely be reluctant to decline the requested relief. And the woman who endangers her baby from refusal to follow apparently sensible medical advice is an unappealing defendant whose judgment is in doubt. Moreover, the great majority of women involved in such suits are poor minority mothers, and a large proportion are unmarried and do not speak English. Such facts may encourage the judge to believe that the mother simply does not understand the medical advice she was given, and that her refusal of care is thus not truly informed.

On the other hand, Caesarean sections are major surgery, despite the declining maternal mortality rate, and one can find no examples other than the Caesarean section cases in which one person is legally compelled to undergo surgery for the benefit of another. So if we analogize to other issues, we find that even where the child's death is the almost certain outcome of maternal refusal to submit to a Caesarean section, and, even if we treat the unborn

child as having all the moral claims of a fully
instated person, compelling Caesareans is virtually
unprecedented.

The unborn child is of course fully dependent on
his mother's decision; no one else can help him. But
while that fact may make her refusal morally repug-
nant, it still provides no warrant for coercing cooperation in the law. Consider, for example, the analogous and tragic case of McFall v. Shimp, 10 Pa.
D.C.3d 90 (1978), in which the plaintiff was fatally
ill with aplastic anemia. His only hope was a bone
marrow transplant, and Shimp, a cousin, was the
only member of his family whose marrow was sufficiently compatible to be a donor. Shimp refused.
Bone marrow extraction is a painful process, but it
is clearly less risky to the donor than major surgery
such as a Caesarean section. McFall brought this
action seeking to compel the life-saving marrow
donation from his cousin, but the court turned him
down. Although it found Shimp's conduct morally
reprehensible, it concluded that to require him to
donate marrow "would change every concept and
principle upon which our society is founded.... For
a society which respects the rights of one individual,
to sink its teeth into the ... neck of one of its
members and suck from it sustenance for another
member, is revolting to our hard-wrought concepts
of jurisprudence." This line drawn at bodily invasion is a familiar one. For example, it is well established, even in the criminal law, that one cannot
compel a witness to undergo surgery or, for exam-

ple, to have his stomach pumped, in order to provide access to critical evidence.

Of course a parent's obligation to his or her child is greater than a cousin's, and so we can surely require more of a mother than a cousin. But it is still doubtful that we can require submission to surgery. There is certainly no precedent, for example, for compelling an unwilling mother to donate bone marrow, or an organ. Such cases would of course be rare—parents and siblings are generally willing to make such donations, just as pregnant women are generally willing to deliver by Caesarean section where that is necessary for their child. The closest case involving a parent is probably Application of George, 630 S.W.2d 614 (Mo.App.1982), involving an adult adoptee who needed medical information from his biological parents in order to identify compatible bone marrow donors essential to the treatment of his leukemia. A blood test of his father was critical. The petitioner's father was identified in the confidential adoption records, and he was located by the trial judge. He refused to cooperate, denying that he was in fact the father. The trial judge went to great lengths to persuade him to submit to a blood test; it was clear that the judge believed strongly that this man should cooperate. But when he refused no order was entered and his identity was not disclosed to the applicant.

More recent appellate authority is in accord with this analysis. In Baby Boy Doe, 632 N.E.2d 326 (Ill.App.1994), a woman was diagnosed at 35 weeks of pregnancy with a placenta defect that compromised the oxygen supply to her baby. Doctors recommended immediate delivery by Caesarean section, which she rejected on the basis of her "personal religious beliefs". The County Attorney filed a wardship petition, but the court sustained the mother. It did not rely on her vague religious objection, but rather held more generally that a competent woman's choice to refuse a medical procedure "as invasive as a cesarean section" must be honored, even if the choice will harm her fetus. The court rejected any balancing of the mother's interests against the fetus', and distinguished earlier cases involving blood transfusions on the ground that, as compared to Caesarean sections, such transfusions are "relatively non-invasive and risk-free".

On one level the distinction is apt, particularly as the objecting women in cases like *Jefferson* and *Raleigh–Fitkin* in fact oppose the transfusion and not the surgery. On the other hand, the distinction is irrelevant if one believes that a blood transfusion is still a bodily invasion which the mother has an absolute right to resist, without regard to any balancing of fetal interests. And in fact a later Illinois decision reached this conclusion, holding that blood transfusions could not be ordered over the objection of a Jehovah's Witness, then about 35 weeks' pregnant, despite medical evidence that transfusions were the only available treatment that would raise her hemoglobin levels. The doctors testified that if her hemoglobin levels were not raised, both she and

her baby had only a 5% chance of survival. In re
Brown, 689 N.E.2d 397 (Ill.App.1997).

Is any procedure sufficiently benign that it may
be imposed on an unwilling pregnant woman when
necessary to protect her child's health? We consider
that question more fully below, in Section 2. The
precedent we have examined certainly suggests,
however, that fetal surgery—available since 1982 at
a few specialized medical centers—could not be
carried out over the pregnant's woman's objection.
That procedure allows the repair of certain medical
problems of the developing child, such as a blocked
bladder, in-utero, thus avoiding irreversible damage
which the condition might otherwise bring about.

The law's apparent resolution of the Caesarean
section question is unsatisfying to many. This is
particularly true because most people—and certainly most pregnant women—believe pregnant woman
should agree to reasonable medical procedures truly
important to protecting the developing child's
health. And indeed, many who work in hospital
obstetric departments believe that in nearly all
cases in which consent is not initially forthcoming,
it can be obtained through better communication
with the pregnant woman. What is usually needed
is not coercion, but personnel sensitive to the woman's cultural traditions and fluent in her native
language, able to successfully counsel her to consent. But even if this point is generally true, there
will still be some with religious or other objections
who are not responsive to such counseling. Ultimately, then, this may be a case in which we must

distinguish the moral conclusion from the legal rule. Even if we believe it is morally wrong for a woman to refuse consent to a standard medical procedure reasonably thought necessary for her fetus' health, we may also believe that there is no acceptable remedy the law may provide to coerce the woman who is unwilling. Suppose she defies the court order? Should medical personnel be authorized to restrain her forcibly to carry out the procedures over her objection? Most find that prospect distasteful, at least.

It is nonetheless not unprecedented. In *Brown, supra,* the trial court had ordered the contested transfusion, which was carried out before the appellate decision reversing the trial court's order. The court reported that the doctors "yelled at and forcibly restrained, overpowered and sedated" the objecting patient. In *Baby Boy Doe, supra,* the public guardian and physician, apparently unwilling to attempt a Ceasarean section under such conditions, did not actually seek an order authorizing the operation over the mother's objections. They instead asked the court to provide that she could be held in contempt if the baby was born either dead or severely retarded as a result of her refusal. Consider whether the threat of contempt is likely to alter the behavior of a woman who has not responded to a careful explanation of why her decision itself poses these very risks for her child.

The difficulty of designing an acceptable remedy in the Caesarean cases is accompanied by a concern that legal coercion may ultimately harm more children than it helps. This concern was one reason for the previously quoted policy statement of the American College of Obstetricians and Gynecologists. In discouraging legal action, ACOG considered not only the pregnant woman's immediate autonomy claims, but also the more general impact of such legal actions on medical practice. By resorting to legal action to enforce their advice, physicians may not only risk destroying their relationship with that particular patient, but may also discourage others from seeking medical assistance. More babies might therefore suffer from a rule allowing coerced Caesareans, than if legal action is foregone in those rare cases in which medical personnel cannot persuade the mother to consent.

2. Fetally Toxic Maternal Behavior During Pregnancy

If the law cannot compel a woman to undergo surgery for the benefit of her developing child, can it require her to avoid drugs and alcohol, to stop smoking, or to eat a healthy diet? Can it require her husband or partner to avoid smoking in her presence? On one hand, such requirements impose no bodily intrusion and no risk to her health. On the other hand, they do require unusually intrusive regulation of personal conduct that in some cases is otherwise lawful.

Arguably, the most appropriate legal tool for such intrusion is the civil child abuse and neglect law. It is intended to protect children, and the ultimate remedy ordinarily is removal of the child from the parents' custody, a step often taken when the child cannot otherwise be protected. It is often hoped that parents will alter their conduct to avoid such removal. Direct orders regulating parental conduct are less common. But when the fetus is our concern, the threat of removal may prove less helpful. Removal after the child's birth is in principle available, and has sometimes been used, as many states treat conduct during pregnancy to be within the scope of child protective statutes. But see Pima Cty. Juvenile Severance Action S–120171, 905 P.2d 555 (Ariz.App.1995) (fetal abuse cannot be the basis for termination of parental rights). But post-birth removal cannot reverse the harm done to the child during the pregnancy, and thus does not address the problem unless it serves to deter the pregnant woman from fetally toxic behavior. It may deter some, but clearly not all. Is any other remedy possible? Can one effectively regulate maternal behavior during pregnancy? Can one incarcerate the recalcitrant pregnant woman to compel her compliance? Should one? These are the questions we address here.

There is surely no doubt that the problem is serious. Consider alcohol abuse. Medical experts have estimated that drinking by pregnant women harms about 2 in 1,000 fetuses and is a leading cause of mental retardation. On the Pine Ridge Indian Reservation in South Dakota, approximately 25 percent of the children were born with fetal alcohol syndrome, which can have devastating and permanent effects on a child's development. Tribal

elders, in a desperate effort to protect the children
as well as the Tribe's future, locked up one woman
during her pregnancy to keep her from drinking. *A
New Toll of Alcohol Abuse,* N.Y. Times, July 19,
1989, at page 1.

Or consider drug abuse. A 1988 survey of selected
hospitals found wide differences among them in the
proportion of addicted mothers, but the data from
some hospitals was quite startling. For example, at
a hospital in Sacramento affiliated with the University of California, urine tests of pregnant women,
taken during labor, found that 25 percent showed
evidence of cocaine, amphetamine, or heroin use.
Similar results were found at hospitals in Boston,
New York, and Delaware during the late 1980s. The
risk to the child is serious. Prenatal cocaine exposure can cause seizures after birth, premature birth,
retarded fetal growth, various structural abnormalities in the genitals and urinary organs, and prenatal
strokes, which in turn may result in lasting brain
damage.

The law's experience with maternal drug addic-
tion predates modern cocaine abuse. For many
years some states have ruled that the child of a
narcotic addict is per se an abused child, and therefore allow removal of the child from the mother at
birth. Others hold specifically that harm caused the
child during pregnancy by the mother's heroin ad-
diction can be the basis of a neglect finding. In some
states, standards for the termination of parental
rights have been expanded to specifically include
drug dependency which the parent has failed to

have treated successfully. These laws sometimes distinguish criminal drug abuse from non-criminal behavior posing similar risks on children. For example, the New York Social Services Department, in an administrative proceeding, held that a child abuse report cannot be established by evidence that the mother drank excessively. In re D.W., 10 Fam. L.Rep. 1359 (B.N.A.1984). But not always. See Fla. Stat. Ann. § 415.503(9)(a) (West Supp. 1997), treating drugs and alcohol alike ("use by the mother of a controlled substance or alcohol during pregnancy, when the child, demonstrably adversely affected by such usage" constitutes "harm" to child).

But of course a rule that drug abuse during pregnancy may support a finding of child neglect after birth does not address the irreversible damage that those undeterred by the rule will cause their child during pregnancy. In some cases, of course, pregnant substance abusers who seek help may find no treatment program available to them. But in other cases the problem is will, not way. Consider, e.g., Angela M.W. v. Kruzicki, 561 N.W.2d 729 (Wis. 1997). Angela's obstetrician suspected her of cocaine abuse. He confronted her with blood test findings and counseled her to enroll in an inpatient drug treatment program. Her response was to cease coming for pre-natal care. He then reported her to county authorities, who relied upon child abuse statutes to obtain a court order allowing them to take "custody of the fetus"—and thus custody of Angela—if she did not remain in a treatment facility. The order was reversed by a divided Wisconsin

Supreme Court, which held that Angela's fetus was not a "child" within the meaning of the relevant state statute. They did not rule on whether such a remedy would be constitutional if the legislature provided it.

Efforts to address the issue through the criminal law rather than the civil child abuse laws have also met with limited success. One must observe that the policy goal of these prosecutions is unclear. The cases are generally brought after disaster has already struck, so that no remedial purpose is possible, unless one believes some general deterrence will be achieved. The Supreme Court of Florida reversed the conviction of Jennifer Johnson, whose child was born with traces of cocaine in its blood. *Johnson v. State*, 602 So.2d 1288 (Fla.1992). The prosecutor argued unsuccessfully that Ms. Johnson violated the criminal law by "delivering" cocaine to her child via the umbilical cord, during the 1½ minutes between the emergence of the child's head from the birth canal (after which it was a "child" and not a "fetus") and the clamping of the cord. The Court held the statute was not intended by the the legislature to apply to such facts. Prosecutions in other states brought on *Johnson* theory have met the same fate.

The principal exception to this pattern is Whitner v. State, 492 S.E.2d 777 (S.C.1997), which sustained the application of a criminal child endangerment statute to a woman's ingestion of crack cocaine during the third trimester of her pregnancy, holding that a viable fetus is a "person" within the meaning

of that statute. An earlier California case, heavily
publicized at the time, went the other way on
similar charges. That prosecution of Pamela Rae
Monson for violation of a statute making it a misde-
meanor to "willfully omit ... to furnish necessary"
medical care to one's child ended in a dismissal, on
the grounds that the statute had not been intended
to apply to prenatal acts or omissions. Ms. Monson
was charged with ignoring her physician's advice to
stop using amphetamines and marijuana for the
remainder of her pregnancy and to seek immediate
medical assistance if she began to hemorrhage. Her
child, born with massive brain damage, died at six
weeks.

Should pregnant drug abusers be placed in some
form of involuntary confinement if necessary, to
protect their fetus—hopefully, in well-run treatment centers? On the practical level the principal
objection is that such a program would be ineffective, or even harmful, because the affected women,
like Angela M.W., would in consequence avoid prenatal care, and otherwise try to keep themselves
from coming to the authorities' attention. That
argument is plausible but hard to evaluate. If real
effort and resources were put into enforcement, and
into creating proper placements for those affected,
it might perhaps succeed. Should it? Did the Pine
Ridge Reservation elders have it right?

There are of course potential constitutional issues. Consider *People v. Pointer,* 199 Cal.Rptr. 357
(App.1984). The defendant mother was convicted of
criminal child endangerment as a consequence of

her fanatical insistence that her two small children adhere exclusively to a macrobiotic diet that had brought one of them near death. She remained unrelenting throughout, even endangering the sicker one by covertly breast feeding him in the hospital, in violation of the physician's explicit instructions (her own diet made her milk dangerous to the child in his weakened state). She fled with her children to Puerto Rico at one point, in an ultimately unsuccessful effort to evade the authorities and continue her children on the disputed diet. Faced with these facts and others that persuaded him that the defendant would endanger any future children as well, the trial judge imposed, as a condition of her probation, a requirement that she not conceive. A sympathetic court of appeals reluctantly overruled this order, concluding that while its purpose was "salutary" it nonetheless unconstitutionally burdened the defendant's privacy rights by effectively requiring her to obtain an abortion if she became pregnant, or have her probation revoked.

Yet the appeals court explained its conclusion in part by urging, as an alternative and presumably acceptable condition, that Pointer be tested periodically for pregnancy and that if she became pregnant she be required to follow an intensive "prenatal and neonatal treatment program monitored by both the probation officer and by a supervising physician." It then remanded to the trial court to allow it to fashion such an alternative set of conditions. The appeals court in *Pointer* thus offered, as the acceptable alternative, the very kind of pregnancy regulation that many would question as excessively intrusive. In *Pointer* such monitoring could presumably be imposed as a condition of probation. Would it be less burdensome on the defendant's privacy than simply requiring her to remain unpregnant? Would it be any more practical to enforce?

These and related questions may seem particularly relevant in considering how to deal with drug-abusing pregnant women. Because drug abuse is typically criminal apart from their pregnancy, lawmakers have more constitutional leeway in deciding how to deal with them. Some report that trial judges often use their sentencing discretion to incarcerate pregnant women convicted of drug abuse—or sometime, of other crimes, if they are also drug users—for a period at least long enough to bring them to their due date, even if nonpregnant offenders might receive lesser sentences or even probation. Involuntary assignment to a drug treatment program, as was attempted in *Angela,* seems preferable, and certainly more straightforward. It is perhaps ironic that while constitutional issues might be more easily avoided if pregnant drug abusers are confined pursuant to the criminal rather than civil law, the civil law may be both a more effective and more humane tool.

There is nonetheless the legitimate fear that civil regulation initially aimed at behavior constituting criminal drug abuse might end up casting a wider net. It could easily extend beyond controlled substances to abuse of alcohol, an extension many would surely urge. But then, is confinement also appropriate to suppress occasional alcohol consumption, or chain smoking? Few would go that far, but what can be offered as the limiting principle? One relevant consideration is the state of the scientific evidence. Suppose available evidence supports claims that heavy drinking during pregnancy has a high probability of causing specifically identified problems, while the harm risked by smoking is less well-identified, and less likely to occur. Scientific evidence might also bear upon the intrusion necessary to forestall the harm. For example, as neuroscientists learn more about the development of the brain in-utero, they may be able to pinpoint specific windows of fetal vulnerability to exposure to particular toxic agents. Suppose, for example, we learned that the damage caused by alcohol abuse could be avoided almost entirely if no alcohol is consumed between the 13th and 16th weeks of pregnancy? Perhaps regulation pinpointed at this vulnerable period could be justified where more wide-ranging regulation would not be.

For the most part such possibilities lie in a future world with more certain scientific information. But the questions can be put most clearly by examining one particular example that has received attention in the literature, which presents a useful paradigm for testing our beliefs on these questions. PKU is a congenital enzyme deficiency rendering the infant incapable of metabolizing phenylalanine. At one time children born with this defect became severely retarded, but this result is now avoided through a mass screening program on all newborns. Affected infants are placed on special diets. The traditional medical understanding has been that they need not continue the diet after reaching physical maturity, because their continued inability to metabolize phenylalanine causes no difficulties in adults. (Very recent scientific research casts some doubt on this traditional view, suggesting the diet may aid the cognitive functioning of PKU adults as well, but for purpose of this discussion we may ignore this development.) In recent years women born with PKU who benefitted from neonatal screening programs have now reached adulthood and become pregnant themselves. These now-pregnant former PKU babies must resume the limited diet of their childhood, not for their benefit, but to avoid disastrous consequences for their baby. While the unmetabolized phenylalanine in the mother causes her little harm, it apparently crosses the placenta in such amounts that it overwhelms even a normal baby's capacity to deal with it. The result is severe retardation, an abnormally small head, congenital heart disease, and other difficulties. There is no effective treatment after birth for most of the baby's problems.

There is, however, a simple, effective, and risk-free program that allows the PKU mother to shield her baby from this fate. She must, during pregnancy, go back on the low phenylalanine diet she ate as a child. She can eat some normal foods, in carefully controlled amounts—breads, cereals, fruits, vegetables. But her main source of protein is a specially prepared paste of L-amino acids to which vitamins, minerals, carbohydrates and fats have been added. This paste tastes bad, and the mother's access to normal foods is restricted. But if she keeps to this diet during her pregnancy her child has the same prospect of health as other children. If she does not, her child will suffer irremediable, and possibly catastrophic, abnormalities. If the mother were to refuse to comply with her physician's advice to adhere to this diet, should a judge be empowered to order her to comply?

Some commentators argue such direct coercive sanctions can be justified only if the intrusion is minimal and would avoid a severe handicap in the child that physicians were very confident would otherwise occur. An example might be case in which the needed treatment requires only a one-time intervention of minimal risk to the mother, such as a single administration of a drug of known safety. Effective intervention with the PKU mother, however, would involve long-term incarceration and control over her diet. Moreover, it seems unlikely that allowing this kind of remedy could in fact help the child of the recalcitrant PKU mother, since by the time one would have the evidence necessary to establish the need for intervention, she would have already doomed her child by departing from the necessary diet.

Other writers see any efforts to intervene in the pregnancy as but another example of gender-based restrictions on women's autonomy. Certainly, any policy allowing increased impositions on a pregnant woman's autonomy to aid her unborn child must be part of a larger, gender-neutral policy that reaches men as well. For instance, men might be compelled either parent to donate blood, or possibly bone marrow, to their born child if necessary to save the child's life or prevent substantial harm. Thus, even though pregnancy is unique to women, a principle that would allow us to sometimes intervene in pregnancy could apply to men as well. But this would cast in doubt cases like McFall v. Shimp, and it involves only a one time intervention, not long term coercive incarceration.

For now these questions have no clear legal answer. It seems likely, however, that in future years new medical knowledge will allow them to be put in more compelling forms.

INDEX

References are to Pages

458 *INDEX*
References are to Pages

†